PARALYZING SUMMER

PARALYZING SUMMER

The True Story of the Ann Arbor
V.A. Hospital Poisonings and Deaths

ZIBBY ONEAL

AND

S. MARTIN LINDENAUER

UNIVERSITY OF MICHIGAN PRESS
Ann Arbor

Published in the United States of America by the
University of Michigan Press
Manufactured in the United States of America
♾ Printed on acid-free paper

2019 2018 2017 2016 4 3 2 1

A CIP catalog record for this book is available from the British Library.

Library of Congress Cataloging-in-Publication Data

Names: Oneal, Elizabeth, author. | Lindenauer, S. Martin, author.
Title: Paralyzing summer : the true story of the Ann Arbor V.A. Hospital poisonings and deaths / Elizabeth Oneal and S. Martin Lindenauer.
Description: Ann Arbor : University of Michigan Press, 2016.
Identifiers: LCCN 2016013652| ISBN 9780472053216 (pbk. : alk. paper) | ISBN 9780472073214 (hardcover : alk. paper) | ISBN 9780472122295 (e-book)
Subjects: LCSH: Narciso, Filipina Bobadilla, 1946– | Perez, Leonora, 1944– | Murder—Michigan—Ann Arbor—Case studies. | Poisoning—Michigan—Ann Arbor—Case studies. | Veterans Administration Hospital (Ann Arbor, Mich.)
Classification: LCC HV6534.A395 O54 2016 | DDC 364.152/3092—dc23
LC record available at https://lccn.loc.gov/2016013652

CONTENTS

PREFACE

This book details a series of mysterious poisonings suffered by patients at the Ann Arbor Veterans Administration Hospital, an affiliated hospital of the University of Michigan Health System, during the summer of 1975. Every effort has been made to report these events as they occurred and without bias or conjecture. The book is based on personal interviews and the recollections of participants, as well as newspaper accounts and court records. For the sake of anonymity, the names of patients involved in these events have been altered. The identities of all others in this story remain unchanged in the text.

PART 1

THE INVESTIGATION

CHAPTER 1

The Veterans Administration Hospital

ANN ARBOR, MICHIGAN

1975

It was a Saturday afternoon late in July. In the Veterans Administration Hospital (VA) aides on the wards were collecting lunch trays. A few patients in wrinkled cotton robes were shuffling slowly in the halls. It seemed that the hospital was settling in for a quiet afternoon when suddenly red emergency lights began flashing high on corridor walls throughout the building. Doctors' pagers began to shrill, announcing the need for immediate help. In the Intensive Care Unit (ICU) on the hospital's third floor a patient had suddenly stopped breathing.

Moments earlier a male nurse, glancing across the eight beds in the unit's open ward, had seen that a patient by the name of Leonard Meadows was in distress. The man lay thrashing, shaking, gasping for air. His face was an ashen gray. The nurse started toward him. The man collapsed. Before the nurse could reach his bed, the man had stopped breathing.

If the nurse had had time to wonder, he might have questioned why a patient who had seemed in stable condition a half hour earlier should suddenly be in such distress, but there was no time to wonder. Shouting an alert, he rushed to do what he could.

Feeling for any obstruction in the man's throat, and finding none, the nurse thrust back the man's jaw, clamped a plastic mask over his nose and mouth, and began to pump air manually into his lungs, using a device known medically as an ambu-bag. Working like a bellows, the bag expressed air as the nurse compressed it. Steadily, repeatedly, he compressed it, knowing that ambu-bagging was, at best, a stopgap measure, a way to supply vital oxygen until a doctor arrived to begin an intubation. Anxiously the nurse glanced toward the unit's doorway. With relief he saw that help was already rushing in.

A Code 7 alert is a call to all available medical personnel anywhere in the hospital to respond without delay. The speed of the response is impressive. Within minutes of the summons interns and residents, medical students and nurses were racing toward the ICU. Minutes later they were crowding into the narrow space around the patient's bed. A nurses' aide came dodging between them, pushing a cart stocked with equipment that would be needed for an intubation. A respiratory therapist hurried into the room and, moving the patient's intravenous (IV) rack to one side, trundled a mechanical ventilator into place beside the bed.

Jon Benner, a resident from the surgical service, went to work at once. Bending over the motionless patient, he began the necessary procedure. Into the man's throat he inserted a laryngoscope. This battery-lighted, metal-bladed instrument would serve to make way for the thin, plastic endotracheal tube that he intended to slip between the man's vocal cords and then into his windpipe. Once in place and connected to the ventilator, the tube would carry oxygen directly into the man's lungs for as many hours as this was needed.

Quickly, with the help of the lighted scope, Benner eased the tube into place. The therapist reached for the free end of the tube and attached it to the ventilator. The ventilator wheezed into action. The man's chest began to rise and fall.

Within two or three minutes it was evident to those standing around the bed that the resuscitation was having an effect. Although the man lay limp and unmoving, it was clear that the ventilator was forcing air into his lungs. His normal color was returning.

This was a quick response and one that surprised Benner. It was not typical of most of the breathing arrests he had witnessed. Ordinarily eight or ten minutes might elapse before a patient undergoing an arrest began to respond to resuscitation if, in fact, he or she responded at all. Patients suffering breathing arrests were almost always very ill. Often in these cases resuscitation failed, the illness engendering the arrest having overwhelmed all efforts to reverse the process. To Benner, Meadows's swift response seemed a curious exception.

Meadows was a sixty-one-year-old retired farmer who had undergone surgery the day before to remove a malignant tumor from his right lung. The surgeons felt that the procedure had been successful. Postoperatively Meadows had been recovering satisfactorily. On the morning following the surgery, Dr. Kalia Sadasivan, a surgical resident who had assisted at the procedure, spent fifteen or twenty minutes talking with Meadows and reported that he seemed to be in good condition.

Sadasivan remembered starting home that afternoon, sure that Meadows was doing well, but when he arrived his telephone was ringing, the hospital calling to tell him Meadows was in arrest. "I didn't believe it," Sadasivan said. "I said, 'Please check to make sure it is Mr. Meadows and not someone else.' I'd spoken to the man hardly ten minutes prior to the phone call." When he returned to the hospital, he found Meadows already intubated.

The next day Dr. Anne Hill, the head of anesthesiology at the hospital, was astonished to learn of Meadows's arrest. "I couldn't believe it when they told me," she said. "He was in great shape after surgery. I could see no reason for the arrest."

Hill, a small, red-haired, Irish-born woman, was known in the hospital as a doctor who showed unusual concern for the patients she had anesthetized for surgery, paying close attention to their condition and recovery for days after the surgery was completed. Meadows was one of these patients, and his arrest troubled her a good deal.

There were none of the underlying problems that might cause such an event to occur, she explained later. The surgery itself could cause shortness of breath but not a complete cessation of breathing. There was no evidence of a heart problem to explain the episode. Meadows's pulse was reported strong throughout the resuscitation, and an electrocardiogram showed nothing unusual. Subsequent scans revealed no blood clot or other unexpected abnormality in his lungs; there had been no obstruction in his throat and no problem inserting the laryngoscope. In fact that had been easy, Benner reported. He had encountered no resistance to the instrument, no spasm or gagging as would be expected. It was almost as though the muscles in Meadows's throat were paralyzed, which was puzzling in itself. "And why did he recover so quickly?," Hill wondered. None of this was typical of a breathing arrest caused by underlying illness. There appeared to be no obvious explanation for any part of the event.

On Sunday morning, the twenty-seventh, the doctors removed Meadows's breathing tube. His seeming paralysis had disappeared, and he had no trouble breathing on his own. He ate normally and was able to leave his bed and walk a little in the unit later that day. Apparently he was suffering no serious aftereffects from the arrest the day before. All seemed to have been resolved and was going well for him until shortly after five o'clock, when he stopped breathing for a second time.

Hillary Stitt, whose husband Gordon was lying in a nearby bed, was the first to see that Meadows was in trouble. As she recalled later, "He was throwing his arms and legs around and kind of short of breath like a person that had been running. . . . His wife had just left, and I thought, my goodness, I hope there isn't anything really wrong with him because when she left she thought he was getting along fine. But he was heaving like he couldn't breathe. So I said, 'Oh my God, I'd better get somebody.'" She ran to find a nurse.

Dr. Sadasivan was on the ninth floor when his pager sounded, signaling another crisis in the ICU. He started for the unit at once, running down the flights of stairs to the third floor, where he joined others rushing into the room. As Mrs. Stitt recalled later, "it was like people were coming out of the woodwork."

Feeling for a pulse in the carotid artery in Meadows's neck and finding one, Sadasivan determined that this was no heart problem and began an intubation. But again there seemed to be no obvious reason for the arrest and nothing to explain its sudden onset. That Meadows had arrested twice in just over twenty-four hours and for no apparent reason either time was more than troubling. But his was only the beginning of the mysterious arrests that day. A few hours later Gordon Stitt stopped breathing.

Mrs. Stitt, leaving the hospital earlier that evening, had thought her husband was doing fine, just as Mrs. Meadows had. She was astonished when, sometime after ten o'clock, the hospital called to tell her that he had stopped breathing. Returning to the ICU, she found her husband intubated and unable to speak because of the apparatus in his mouth and throat connecting him to a ventilator. "And the doctors couldn't tell me why it had happened," she said. The doctors didn't know.

Stitt had undergone surgery a few days earlier to repair an aneurysm, an abnormal enlargement of the aorta, in his abdomen. This had been a significant procedure but not one that would be expected to give rise to a breathing arrest. The doctors agreed on that. Stitt's arrest was baffling.

At 9:45 the following evening Stitt arrested again. Fifteen minutes later Homer Mercer, an elderly patient in a nearby bed, was found blue and struggling to breathe.

This was five arrests in three days. In the next three days there were six more, three in the ICU and three on other floors. None could be satisfactorily explained.

Prior to the summer of 1975, hospital statistics show that the number of arrests occurring anywhere in the hospital in the space of a month was approximately eight, or two per week. In the last six days of July 1975 there were eleven.

So began the nightmare that was to engulf the hospital that summer, a nightmare that would lead eventually to media coverage coast to coast, to a hospital in turmoil, to a community in uproar, and ultimately to a trial for multiple murders.

CHAPTER 2

From its beginnings in 1953 the Ann Arbor VA, as it is usually called, has maintained a close relationship with the University of Michigan Medical Center, located a mile or two away across the Huron River. Medical students, interns, and resident physicians in training at the university spend several months' rotation at the VA as part of that training in surgery, internal medicine, and related subspecialties. The hospital's senior staff, responsible for the supervision and instruction of these young doctors, is comprised of physicians from the University of Michigan Medical School faculty. They head the hospital's various departments, or services as they are called.

The hospital is proud of its university affiliation. The patients benefit, it is believed, from the large number of young doctors available to attend them. And it is these doctors-in-training, or house staff members as they are called, who undertake the day-to-day patient care.

For these young doctors the day begins early. Often before patients' breakfast trays have arrived on the floors, they are making their rounds, visiting the patients in their care. In groups organized by specialty, they snake through the wards in their white coats, stopping to gather at patients' bedsides. Students, who have yet to earn their MD degrees, and interns, who have only recently been awarded theirs, stand listening and learning as the residents speak to patients. It is the residents, many of them in their fourth and fifth years of postgraduate training, who make decisions about the patients' care and treatment in consultation with members of the senior staff.

By seven-thirty on weekday mornings, rounds finished, the residents on the surgical service will be scrubbed and ready to enter the operating rooms. Residents on the internal medicine service head for the clinics to evaluate the problems and complaints of the many outpatients scheduled to be seen that day. Toward evening the groups will assemble again to make another tour of their patients, stopping to speak with families to answer questions and explain treatments. It is a long day.

For some the day is longer still. On a rotating basis one resident from the surgical service and one from internal medicine join forces to take night duty. After the halls are emptied of visitors, the patients are settled in for the night, and the lights in the corridors are dimmed, these two will remain on call, responsible for whatever problems or emergencies may arise until eight o'clock the next morning.

Traditionally, on the first day of July a changeover in the house staff occurs. A new group of students, interns, and residents arrives to replace those finishing their VA rotation. On the first day of July 1975 approximately sixty new doctors and students took over from those who were leaving. Before they had been at the hospital long, many would witness one or more of the mysterious breathing arrests that were beginning to occur in increasing numbers as July gave way to August.

The more junior members of the house staff seem not to have realized how unusual these numbers were. Dr. Michael McLeod, who was an intern that summer, said, "I had no context for how often they [the arrests] normally happened. Maybe I was naive, but I thought this was just the way things were at the VA." Those with more experience knew better. The numbers *were* unusual they agreed. "But the patients had all kinds of problems," one doctor remembered, "so we thought maybe that was enough to explain the arrests, their age and their general poor health."

A great many of the patients in the hospital that summer *were* elderly. Many were veterans of World War II, men who had spent their working lives as farmers, mechanics, or laborers on construction crews or the assembly lines in the auto plants near Detroit. Most were men of small means who felt lucky to have access to the VA and the care they received there at the government's expense.

Bart Martin had been a carpenter. Now retired and in his seventies, he was being monitored for a heart problem in the three-bed Cardiac Care Unit (CCU) adjacent to the ICU's open ward. On the twenty-ninth of July, at about six-thirty in the evening, he was finishing his supper, sitting up in bed with his feet on the floor, a nurses' aide recalled. A few minutes later, glancing toward him, she saw that he had collapsed and was struggling to breathe.

Roberta Kurtz was one of the new interns on the internal medicine service that summer. On the twenty-ninth she was having supper with a colleague in the canteen on the third floor. Musak was playing softly in the room. The two had just begun to eat when her companion's pager sounded a Code 7. Trouble in the ICU. Her companion jumped up from the table, and, leaving the food behind, Kurtz followed him down the hall and into the unit. There she found Martin in arrest, a resuscitation team gathered around his bed.

Kurtz couldn't understand this. Martin was a patient she knew well and had visited daily. That afternoon she had spent time chatting with him and had believed he was in good shape. Now he lay motionless. Checking, she could see that his heart was not a problem. His cardiac monitor showed nothing abnormal. Once again the cause was unclear.

In the days following his resuscitation, Martin claimed to remember the entire experience, and this was puzzling, too. Typically, patients suffering respiratory arrests caused by underlying illnesses lose consciousness almost immediately. Martin apparently had not. He remembered trying to call to a nurse near his bed as his vision began to blur. He had heard footsteps and voices around him as he lost the power to move or speak, and, with some annoyance, he recalled that a member of the resuscitation team had called him an old man. Improbably Martin had been conscious throughout the episode. As the days went by and the arrests continued, patients' failure to lose consciousness became one more baffling aspect of these increasingly baffling events.

Martin was not the only patient to arrest on the evening of the twenty-ninth. Between nine and ten-thirty there were two more arrests in the ICU and two more hurried resuscitations. It seemed to the nurses on duty that night that the emergencies were almost epidemic.

At nine o'clock Homer Mercer arrested for a second time. At ten-thirty the patient arresting was Arthur Lenz. Although Mercer was a man of eighty-seven, Lenz was only forty-six. His arrest seemed to belie the theories that blamed old age for the episodes.

Lenz was an obese man who admitted to having drunk a case of beer a day for thirty years. He had entered the hospital several days earlier suffering severe abdominal pain and almost immediately was taken to the operating room for emergency surgery.

The surgeons found his bowel perforated in at least two places. Cloudy fluid was leaking into his abdominal cavity. To deal with this leakage, the surgeons performed a colostomy, bringing a portion of Lenz's large bowel out through his abdominal wall where they could attach it to a plastic bag to collect the leaking fecal material, preventing infection from spreading within the abdominal cavity.

Postoperatively, Lenz's recovery had not been smooth. The day following the operation the surgeons returned him to the operating room to repair a part of the wound closure that had broken down, but by the twenty-ninth he seemed to be recovering satisfactorily, occupying one of the glass-enclosed isolation rooms in the ICU reserved for patients with infectious conditions. It was in this room, in full view of the nurses at the nurses' station that Lenz went into arrest. As one of the doctors attending him said later, despite what Lenz had been through, and the problems he had had, there was no medical reason to anticipate a breathing arrest. The question of cause remained unanswered.

It was a question that had troubled Anne Hill a good deal since first learning of Leonard Meadows's arrest three days earlier. "It just made no sense to me," she said. "I went down to Intensive Care the day after his arrest and had a look at his chart, but I could find nothing unusual reported. So I spoke to Dr. Sadasivan. I remember I called him at home. I asked, 'Is there anything about Meadows you haven't told me?' He thought about it. He said, 'Well, the nurse told me he was shaking all over just before he stopped breathing.'" Hill paused. "A fever can make a person shake that way, but there was no indication in his chart that Meadows was feverish. The only thing I could think of that might cause such a reaction is a drug called succinylcholine. It's a muscle relaxant, a drug we use in the operating room as an adjunct to anesthesia. It relaxes the muscles in the throat so that the patient won't fight the anesthesia tube going down. The drug can cause shaking."

But succinylcholine had not been ordered for Meadows in the ICU. There was no such order in his chart. "And why would it be?" Hill asked, explaining that succinylcholine is a drug always used in conjunction with a ventilator, since its paralyzing effect on the diaphragm makes spontaneous breathing impossible. "So I thought it couldn't be that," she said.

Yet she remained uneasy. A day or two later she spoke with Dr. Duane Freier, the head of the surgical service. Freier, a fit and wiry Harvard-educated surgeon, was a colleague with whom she had spent many hours in the operating room and much time discussing patients. She told him about Meadows's shaking and her thoughts about succinylcholine. "I wondered whether there could be a mistake in labeling," she said. "Whether maybe something labeled penicillin was in fact succinylcholine."

It seemed a far-fetched idea, they agreed. That all the arresting patients could have received a mislabeled drug was improbable. Still, Hill felt that something needed to be done. She offered to review the charts of the other patients who had arrested in the past several days. "I wanted to look at the charts and see if there was some common factor," she said, "Maybe some other drug had been given to all of them before they arrested."

Freier offered to enlist some help from among the surgery residents to undertake the project, but it seems that Hill proceeded mainly on her own. And, as it turned out, she found few common factors and little that seemed significant apart from the facts that all the patients had had IV fluids running at the time of their arrests and none had received medications just prior to the episodes. At least there were none recorded in their charts.

CHAPTER 3

"Weekend staffing is so unbalanced it is pathetic."

This comment appears in the nursing supervisor's log on a date early in August and is typical of many such entries. A shortage of nurses was a chronic problem in the hospital. To keep the floors adequately staffed was a challenge for the supervisors.

On most floors one registered nurse, with the help of one or two aides, was responsible for as many as thirty patients. Although not all these patients were ill enough to require close monitoring, this was not the case in Intensive Care. There close monitoring was essential, and the shortage of nurses was keenly felt. For some time the ICU nurses had complained about overwork and exhaustion. There were days and nights when they were too busy to stop long enough to have a meal, they said. There was hardly time for them to sit down, and as the number of emergencies multiplied in the last days of July, so did their frustrations and complaints.

Earlier in the year a group of nurses had approached the director of the hospital, Arnold Mouish, with a petition expressing their concerns about understaffing and overwork.

"There is a critical shortage of registered nurses at the Veterans' Hospital," the petition began, then went on to list sixteen areas where understaffing was causing real problems. These ranged from the huge burden of overwork and overtime exhausting the nurses to inadequate and possibly unsafe patient care. It ended with an appeal to the administration to "reevaluate its priorities for nursing service and take appropriate measures to ensure that the number of RN's [registered nurses] at the VA is significantly increased to allow us to practice nursing as we and the professional nursing organization feel we should." The petition was signed by thirty nurses.

In response Mouish directed Gloria Nunley, the chief of nursing, to explain to the signers the facts contributing to the understaffing. Mouish felt that Nunley had not done this adequately.

Lack of money was one of the problems. The funds the US Congress appropriated to serve the nation's veterans hospitals was shared among them according to decisions made by a central authority. In 1975 there were well over one hundred hospitals in the country, and, although the appropriation might have seemed generous in the aggregate, it was not generous when divided more than a hundred ways. This was one reality. Another was the lack of available nurses. Even if funding had not been a problem, finding nurses to hire was *not* an easy undertaking.

Then, as now, too few nurses were being trained in the United States to supply the hospitals that needed them. Most hospitals, seeking to augment their staffs, depended on hiring nurses trained elsewhere. A great number of these nurses came from the Philippines. It is estimated that between 1966 and 1985 twenty-five thousand Filipino nurses immigrated to the United States. The nurses were eager to make the move, seeing it as a positive career choice in terms of both salary and the experience to be gained. The hospitals were eager to employ them, for Filipino nurses were known to be well-trained, conscientious workers. In 1975 the Ann Arbor hospital was one of many in the country employing nurses from the Philippines.

Nunley may have explained the problems, but the petitioning nurses continued to feel that the hospital administration was turning a deaf ear to their very real concerns and failing to give a serious problem serious consideration. The explanation did little to reduce their frustration.

Late in July several ICU nurses decided to try again. The emergencies in the unit were becoming overwhelming. The nurses worried that there were too few of them to adequately respond to the relentless increase and decided to take their concerns to Dr. Freier.

Freier seemed the logical choice. As head of the surgical service he would, of course, be well aware of the number of arrests occurring mainly among the surgery patients. But in addition to this he was soon to take a turn as acting chief of staff, standing in for Dr. Martin Lindenauer, who had been away on sabbatical for several months. In Lindenauer's absence various heads of services had assumed the position. On the first of August Freier was due to take over, and as acting chief he might be in a position to do something about the staffing problem.

Freier had doubtless heard nurses' complaints about overwork and understaffing, which were discussed many times in senior staff meetings. Linking the breathing arrests to the staffing situation may have seemed only a fresh way to give voice to a worn refrain. He may have wondered as well whether the shortage of nurses actually had much to do with the increase in arrests.

In nearly every case the arrests had been discovered quickly and almost always by nurses. Thanks to them the resuscitations had been prompt and unusually successful. Lacking the vigilance of the nurses a far different picture might have emerged. Exhausted though they were, they were not neglecting their patients, and it was difficult to believe that understaffing could be blamed for the problem.

In any case, Freier had little to offer them but sympathy. He said, "I just had absolutely zero comprehension about the money situation, what was available and what wasn't. But I *did* know how hard it was to find nurses. I told them we were always looking for more nurses and that we needed to keep looking. There wasn't much more I could say."

Small consolation this must have been to the worn and worried nurses.

CHAPTER 4

The evening of July 30 was unusually quiet in the ICU. There were not many empty beds in the unit, but there seemed to be no immediate problems. The patients lay in rumpled gowns, most of them asleep under the unit's steady artificial lights. Intravenous fluids dripped in measured quantities into the veins in their arms through plastic tubes attached to the bags that hung on racks beside their beds. Occasionally a patient moaned or muttered incoherently, these sounds mingling with the regular bleeps and wheezes of life support machines, but none seemed in distress.

The main hospital was growing quiet, too. It was past eight o'clock. Visiting hours had ended, and the halls were nearly deserted, only a few nurses moving silently from room to room, checking on their patients. It appeared that this might be a peaceful night.

On the night of the thirtieth the arrests began to move beyond the confines of the ICU. At nine-thirty a patient on the fifth floor arrested. At ten there was a second arrest on 4West and at ten-thirty a third on 4East.

The patient arresting on the fifth floor was Howard Jackson, a seventy-three-year-old double amputee who was suffering from kidney disease, diabetes, and the effects of alcoholism. Clearly his problems were significant, but his doctor, who saw him at the end of the day, believed that his condition had not deteriorated. As the doctor said later, "I thought I would see him alive in the morning."

At just before nine-thirty that evening a nurse stopped to check on Jackson and discovered that his color was bad, his pulse was weak, and he was having trouble breathing. Immediately she ran to call a Code. Almost immediately help began arriving. Yet, in spite of the efforts made to revive him, Jackson did not respond. Doctors pronounced him dead at ten-thirty.

One floor below, on 4West, Daniel Clark lay dozing. He had undergone coronary bypass surgery at University Hospital in June, a procedure not yet performed at the VA because of the prohibitive expense of the necessary equipment. He had been transferred to the VA for his recuperation and that evening was resting comfortably. His wife had left earlier. By nine-thirty he was settled for the night.

But before 10:00 p.m. he woke, gasping. That much he could remember later—gasping, looking at a clock near his bed, and collapsing. A nurses' aide who had come into the room to take his blood pressure saw at once that there was an emergency and hurried to summon help.

A resident who was attending to another patient on 4West heard the call. He went directly to Clark's room, had a look, and ordered a Code. As always, help arrived swiftly. A nurse came running down the hall, pushing a "crash cart," a wheeled vehicle available on every floor stocked with the equipment and medications that might be needed at a resuscitation. She stationed the cart in the hall outside Clark's door. The night nursing supervisor, took charge and began to pass the needed supplies into the room. Doctors started an intubation, and within thirty minutes Clark was stabilized. But almost as soon as this resuscitation ended, a third Code sounded. A patient was arresting on 4East.

This patient, Stuart Neff, a man of sixty, was recovering from surgery for cancer of the bladder. He, too, had been recovering well, well enough that it had seemed unnecessary to keep him in the ICU.

He had been listening to a baseball game when his arrest began, he said. "And I wanted to listen to the game," he told an interviewer later, "but my legs went to sleep, and it wasn't much time before I was asleep clear up to my waist. I was getting groggy."

Through blurring eyes he believed that he saw a nurse just leaving the room. He called to her. "'Nurse! Hey, nurse!' I yelled as loud as I could holler," he said "The last time I hollered I was shaking the bed, and then I passed out."

It is doubtful that Neff "passed out" entirely. One of the cruel aspects of these poisonings was the fact that the patients attacked never lost consciousness completely. Although their bodies lost the ability to function, they remained aware of their situations, able to hear and think and confront the horror of their helplessness but unable to cry out or utter a sound. Neff managed to holler "Nurse!" before he became paralyzed, but few others managed even this much.

To lie so totally helpless must have been a terrifying experience. One patient, who underwent three arrests in August, described the experience as like an instant death. As he reported in a September 1975 interview with the *Detroit Free Press*, "It's like somebody grabbed hold of your throat real quick. And it's just how long you can hold your breath—maybe thirty, maybe sixty seconds. Then your whole body goes numb."

On the night of the thirtieth of July, following his resuscitation, Neff was taken to Intensive Care for observation. He remembered hearing a comment on his way to the ICU that he would repeat later: "I heard a doctor say, 'Boy, the police are sure to be here. This is the third one tonight.'" Possibly this is a comment Neff only imagined having heard when, a few weeks later, the newspapers began to fill with stories about the arrests at the VA. Or perhaps there *was* some talk in the hospital about foul play at that time, although there is nothing to suggest that there was much suspicion yet. On the thirtieth police and poisonings and murder were still the stuff of detective novels. As Jon Benner remembered, "We were looking for all kinds of reasons for these arrests, but foul play wasn't one of them. We weren't thinking of that."

CHAPTER 5

On Saturday, August 2, the temperature was in the nineties. Thunderstorms were forecast for later in the day. At about four o'clock the rain began. Visitors came ducking into the hospital, shaking umbrellas and complaining about the sudden downpour, but by the time visiting hours ended the storm was moving east toward Detroit. There were only faint rumbles of departing thunder to disturb the watery twilight.

A lone security guard, sitting at his desk across from the elevators in the lobby, watched the visitors straggle out. On the floors above the nurses were beginning to dispense evening medications. Again the building was growing quiet, the insistent murmur of television voices drifting through the open doors of patients' rooms and the soft hush of the nurses' rubber-soled shoes the only sounds in the dim corridors.

At nine-fifteen the Codes began. The first one was called for a patient on 4East. At ten-fifteen there was another on 3West. At eleven-fifty a patient arrested in the CCU. In the nursing supervisor's log these August 2 Codes are duly recorded together with the comment, "A terrible nite was had by all."

It was in these early days of August that rumors began to circulate in the hospital. Over coffee in the canteen or in brief moments in the halls there was talk about the unusual number of arrests and speculation about their cause. Some blamed the extremely hot summer weather and the hospital's lack of central air-conditioning, suggesting that the heat could have a debilitating effect on recovering patients. Others wondered whether there could be some problem in the operating room. So many of those arresting were surgery patients; was there contamination in the drugs used there or some problem with the anesthesia?

Dr. Freier and other members of the senior staff had discussed the arrests at length at a meeting on July 30, concluding, as the residents had, that the patients' age and general health were sufficient explanation.

Freier said that until he took over as acting chief of staff on the first of August he had heard about only those arrests occurring among surgery patients. Now, as acting chief, he began to hear about patients who, like Martin, had not undergone surgery. At that point, he said, the extent of the problem really hit home.

In an effort to discover what was going on he asked the Pharmacy and the medical records service to develop a flow sheet of drug information on all patients who had undergone arrests. He consulted with Anne Hill about her chart review and began to review the cases himself. "I spent two agonizing weeks reviewing case after case, trying to resolve the issue [of cause]," he said. "I spent two weeks absolutely wracking my brain with a great deal of angst. It became very obvious that we had not reacted in time."

When the Clinical Executive Board convened for its twice-monthly meeting on August 4, Freier reported that there had been five Code 7s the previous weekend and six on two evenings the preceding week. He reported on the results of Anne Hill's chart review and her discovery that all the arresting patients had had IV fluids running at the time the episodes occurred.

This finding raised the question of contamination. Was the hospital receiving bags containing contaminated fluids from the supplier? Was contamination occurring in the administration or preparation of the IV solutions in the hospital itself?

The doctors discussed the possibility of allergic reactions. They discussed the age and health of the patients once again. Reluctantly they approached the idea that an employee in the hospital was intentionally putting foreign material into the IV bags or the lines running into patients' arms. In that case, they agreed, nurses, Pharmacy personnel, residents, students, in fact almost anyone could be responsible. "But that was unthinkable," Freier said later.

He is quoted in an interview in the *Detroit Free Press* as saying, "I just put it up to them [at the meeting]. I said, 'I'm new at this and I need some advice. Should we go ahead with a formal investigation of all this?'"

Apparently the other members of the board felt such an investigation would be ill-advised, citing adverse publicity and damage to the hospital's reputation. Freier agreed. As he said in a 2007 interview, "Until we put all the numbers together, started making graphs and so forth, to think we could call in the police and say 'we think multiple murders are occurring' was just unthinkable."

In any case, no investigation was undertaken and, as if to vindicate the board's decision, the number of arrests began to decline in the next few days. On August 6 there were two in the ICU. On the eighth there was only one. And then, for the next three days, there appeared to have been none at all anywhere in the hospital. It was as though a siege had lifted.

* * *

On August 12 there were no empty beds in the ICU. In the late afternoon the unit was bustling, aides checking patients' vital signs, residents making rounds and writing orders, nurses going from bed to bed with medications. In the visitors' lounge near the unit a few tired people sat amid a strew of crumpled newspapers and empty soda cans, awaiting their opportunity to spend the short time they were allowed with a patient. One visitor remembered that shortly after six o'clock emergency lights began to flash. The brief respite had ended.

Arthur Lenz was the first patient to arrest that evening, arresting for the second time. At six-twenty Leonard Roberts, a forty-three-year-old projects engineer at Cadillac Motors recovering from bowel surgery, underwent a first arrest, lying in a bed not far from Lenz's isolation room. At seven there was a third.

Thomas Weber, a fifth-year resident in surgery, was in the ICU when Lenz's Code was called. Lenz was a patient Weber knew well. On the day Lenz was admitted in early July, suffering severe abdominal pain, it had been Weber who rushed him to the operating room. He had seen Lenz every day since. Now, hurrying toward the isolation room, he felt puzzled and uneasy. There was no reason that Lenz should arrest. "I knew something strange was going on," Weber said.

On the seventh floor, Dennis Penner, a second-year resident in medicine, was checking on patients when the pager in the pocket of his white coat began to sound. Penner was the medical resident on duty that night, and he wasted no time. Running the stairs to the third floor, he burst through the doors into the ICU and spied Roberts, gasping for breath and pointing to his throat. By the time Penner reached him, Roberts had collapsed and couldn't speak.

As soon as he could, Weber joined Penner at Roberts's bedside, and the two went to work on the resuscitation. To Weber, Roberts appeared to be fully conscious. Although he lay limp, unable to move at all now, his eyes, under half-closed lids, seemed filled with fear. Later this aspect of Roberts's arrest would seem strange and highly suspicious to Weber, but at that moment he had little chance to think about it because, just as Roberts was beginning to respond to the resuscitation, a nurse came hurrying across the unit to announce a third patient in distress.

The third patient was Robert Lippy, a twenty-nine-year-old ex-Marine who was later to describe his arrest as like instant death. Suffering from liver and kidney damage, the result of a shot from a .22 caliber rifle, Lippy was being cared for in a glass-enclosed room adjacent to Lenz's. When Weber and Penner reached him he was lying motionless.

Three arrests in less than an hour and a fourth to follow in forty-five minutes? What was going on? Rushing from one emergency to the next, Weber and Penner had no time to wonder, but later both began to ponder these episodes. Four arrests within two hours was uncommon enough, but the fact that at least three of these seemed to have no obvious cause, that the resuscitations had been relatively easy and the patients had responded quickly—all this made the events stranger still. Weber said, "I was thinking about it at the time, but I was tired." In fact, both Weber and Penner were exhausted.

Because he was the medical resident on duty that night and responsible for whatever might occur, Penner could not take a break and leave the hospital. Weber could, and did briefly, going home long enough to have a meal. When he returned at about nine-thirty his pager began signaling another Code. A patient in a single room on 4East was arresting. Weber ran for the fourth floor.

A nurse met him in the hall. She had discovered the patient, Roy Custer, unresponsive and without a pulse when she entered his room to check his IV. She had called a cardiac arrest at once and begun closed chest massage while she waited for doctors to arrive. "And he was just being treated for a broken hip," she said.

Penner was already at work when Weber entered Custer's room. There were six or eight others in the room as well, but despite the efforts they were making, Custer remained unresponsive, without a pulse, without respirations. Epinephrine, a drug that will typically stimulate the heart to resume functioning, was having no effect. The electrocardiogram remained flat, indicating no movement. There seemed little hope of resuscitation, but the doctors were not giving up.

It was while this ultimately futile struggle to save Custer was still in progress that the next emergency was called. From the hall a nurse cried suddenly, "There's another one in here!" Incredibly it was the patient in the adjoining room. Leaving Custer with the others, Penner and Weber ran the few steps to the neighboring doorway.

The patient in distress appeared to be a young man. His right arm was encased in a white cast that extended from his armpit to his wrist. An intravenous tube sprouted from his left hand. The symptoms he was exhibiting had become all too familiar.

Quickly Weber moved to the head of the bed and began mouth-to-mouth resuscitation while he waited for the instruments he would need for intubation. Penner, in the meantime, was feeling for a pulse in the man's groin. Finding none, he began cardiac massage, pressing both hands down hard on the man's chest, starting a rhythmical compression in hopes of restoring the heart's functioning.

After a few seconds it was clear to Penner that the heart was not responding. "I was getting kind of desperate," he said. "I was afraid the man would die unless I did something fast."

He turned toward the hall and yelled to a student to bring him epinephrine from the crash cart stationed outside the adjoining room. "I was hoping that would do it," he said. The student hurried to provide a syringe filled with the medication. Penner took the syringe and positioned it on the man's chest, finding a space between two ribs. Then he plunged the needle through the chest wall and directly into the heart. Blood spurted into the syringe, propelled by the heart's pressure. Penner injected the epinephrine. Within seconds both doctors could feel a strong and rapid pulse.

The patient, Jeffrey Wallace, was a man in his forties being treated for a fractured elbow suffered when he fell from a ladder while shingling a roof. Although he had struck his right temple when he fell, he claimed never to have lost consciousness. The doctors who examined him initially could find no evidence of a concussion or fracture that might have damaged his brain and would explain the arrest. Wallace had no history of heart problems.

Dr. Booker Wright, the fourth-year orthopedic resident in charge of Wallace's care, was incredulous when a nurse called him at home to report the arrest. By the time he reached the hospital Weber and Penner had nearly finished the resuscitation and Wallace was stabilized, but the question of cause remained unanswered. The doctors stood looking at one another. Wallace's arrest seemed a highly unlikely consequence of a fall that had only fractured an elbow.

A broken hip. A fractured elbow. And the question again: what was going on?

Penner remembered that at about midnight things quieted down. As he was climbing the stairs to the quarters reserved for residents on night duty, hoping for a little sleep, he began to think about a movie he had seen. "It was called *The Hospital,*" he said. "It was about somebody roaming around a hospital, injecting potassium into patients. I guess the possibility was on my mind. I remember thinking how fortunate that every one of the patients had had an IV line in. That's always one of the things at an arrest, you want to get a line in so you can start administering medications to get the heart started. So I thought it was nice they all had lines in already." He thought, too, about how easy the intubations had been and how stable the patients became, "rock stable" he called them, once they were being ventilated. But the possibility of contamination in the intravenous bags troubled him. He worried about other patients in his care, many of whom receiving intravenous fluids.

Still mulling over the arrests, Penner lay down to sleep. "I remember lying in bed and because it was such a crazy night I had the pager right by my ear," he said. "I remember towards morning the pager went off. It was one of these pagers that can give you a verbal message and the beeper went off and the message came: 'Oh my God, a patient went out the window.' I was thinking, 'Okay, I'm dreaming.' And then a minute later I hear there's a cardiac arrest in Admitting. So I'm running down the stairs and then I get to Admitting and someone points out that the arrest is outside. Then it hit me. A patient went out the window. I went outside and here was this dead guy with blood coming out his nose and ears. I looked up and there was a window screen kind of half out on the seventh floor."

The next morning he went to report the night's arrests to his chief, Dr. Ronald Bishop, head of the internal medicine service. Bishop was a soft-spoken, thoughtful man with a professorial demeanor. He had already seen the morning report, which was published each day to inform the heads of services about the events and emergencies of the previous twelve hours. "I hadn't gone over the report as critically as I should," Bishop later told an *Ann Arbor News* reporter. That morning he was preoccupied with the suicide. This took precedence over the arrests Penner was reporting. Most of these, Bishop remembered thinking, could be attributed to age and illness, but the suicide required an inquiry at once.

To Penner, nearly sleepless that morning, the night's events had begun to seem unreal. "Especially that last scene," Penner said, "because it was like five in the morning, dawn, and it's one thing to see a patient in a hospital bed having an arrest. It's another thing to see a dead body outside the hospital on the street."

CHAPTER 6

On that same afternoon, a few hours before the evening's arrests began, Anne Hill had been at University Hospital conferring with Dr. Robert Sweet, the chairman of the Department of Anesthesia and a man she greatly admired. She had consulted him twice before about the situation at the VA. This afternoon she again expressed her uneasiness. Something had to be done, she said. Reasons had to be found for the problem. She was proposing sending a memo to Dr. Freier, urging him to convene a committee to interview the first respondents at each of the arrests, those doctors and nurses who had been at the scene and might provide useful information.

For some time she had been puzzling over the easy intubations the residents reported. As an anesthesiologist she knew that a patient did not ordinarily accept a tube being put down his or her throat without considerable resistance. In the operating room she used a muscle relaxant to counteract this resistance and make it possible to insert an anesthesia tube. How was this possible without a relaxant? She wanted to explore these easy intubations and much else. Interviewing first respondents might yield clues to what was going on, she thought.

Dr. Sweet agreed with her. Action needed to be taken. The next day Hill sent the memo to Freier, suggesting that he form a committee at once.

Hill remembered that she had not been sleeping well for some time. The situation at the hospital was very much on her mind. The rumors she had begun to hear distressed her. But now she had spoken again to Dr. Sweet, had sent the memo to Freier, and felt that she had done what she could. She went to bed that night expecting to sleep better.

It was a sudden terrible certainty that woke her in the night, bringing her fully alert in the darkened bedroom. As she was later to tell an interviewer from the *Detroit News,* "I woke up in the middle of the night and thought suddenly, 'Good God, someone is injecting muscle paralyzing drugs into these people.'"

The next day she went to talk to Dr. Freier about her memo. She hadn't intended to mention her night suspicions, but as she was about to leave his office, "It all just came out," she said, "almost automatically. I told him what I'd thought in the middle of the night about someone injecting these patients with a muscle relaxant."

Freier, of course, remembered this moment. "And I certainly concurred that something really bad was going on, but I thought we should look into it further before we jumped to conclusions." There was no proof, after all, for Hill's suspicions, and the implications were, as Freier said, horrendous.

Jon Benner remembered that early in August some residents began to carry endotracheal tubes with them "to be ready for the next one." Among the nurses in the ICU a sort of grim apprehension had set in. As evening approached they became uneasy. As one nurse described it, "Our eyes were glued to the emergency lights, waiting for them to come on. Before ten-thirty we'd say to each other, 'They [the arrests] are about to begin.'"

By now apprehension was becoming general in the hospital. It seemed that "the next one" could happen anywhere. On any floor, on any ward, in any room a patient might be discovered limp and gasping. Yet, although the arrests were occurring nearly every night, few people recalled suspecting that they were being caused deliberately.

Thomas Weber remembered that after the marathon of resuscitations he performed with Dennis Penner on the night of the twelfth, he grew suspicious. Penner recalled uneasiness as well and remembered his thoughts about the film he had seen earlier. But nearly everyone now, speaking of the arrests that summer, talked about how difficult it was to let themselves believe that there could be someone in their midst deliberately attacking patients.

Some patients, conversely, believed just that. Leonard Roberts, the projects engineer at Cadillac Motors who arrested on the twelfth, claimed to be positive that there was someone trying to kill him.

Arthur Lenz, too, was terrified following the arrests. He begged his sister not to leave him alone in his isolation room, saying he knew a nurse was trying to kill him. "I'm doing all I can [to stay alive]," he told a nephew, "but they're going to kill me." He seemed certain of that.

Such fears may have been, and likely were, discounted as fantasies if they were ever expressed to the doctors and nurses attending these patients. They would have been attributed to illness and drugs and long nights half awake in the ICU. But when an investigation finally began, these fears assumed a new significance.

* * *

There were thirty-one patients on 5East on the fourteenth of August and only one RN and one aide on duty. The aide, questioned later, declared that anyone could have come onto the floor unobserved that night. It seems that someone did.

At twenty-five minutes after ten, Jerry Yost, a patient in a single room on 5East, was found dead in his bed by the nurse on duty. There was no way to know exactly when he had died, she said, but at eight o'clock that evening, when she checked him, he had seemed to be in satisfactory condition. Similarly, Rex Palmer, a patient in a room only two doors farther down the hall, had been judged to be stable and without any significant problems when he was checked earlier. At ten-thirty he was dead.

No Codes were called for Yost and Palmer. Obviously it was too late for that. But the nurse on 5East set about paging the medical doctor on duty, who was needed to pronounce the patients dead for the record. She had a hard time making contact.

Joseph Zibrak, the medical intern on duty that night, was fully occupied in the hospital basement when his pager sounded. He was struggling with a patient who, having escaped from the psychiatry ward, had found his way to the basement and was on a rampage, demanding to leave the hospital and flailing at anyone who tried to get near him. Zibrak and several others had just managed to subdue him when the pager sounded. To have succeeded in subduing the patient was a victory not to be forfeited. Zibrak asked someone else to answer the page.

The night supervisor, Betty Jakim, went to take the call. It was a call from 5East she told him, but it was not an emergency. He could call when he was free.

Fifteen minutes later Zibrak's pager sounded again. Again Jakim answered. She was told that two patients were dead on 5East. Zibrak was upset when he heard this. He couldn't understand why he hadn't been notified that these patients were in critical condition since he was the medical intern on duty that night.

When a patient was critically ill, he explained, the doctor assigned to that patient was responsible for informing the one on night duty about the patient's illness before leaving the hospital for the day. Thus he assumed that the doctor on duty was aware of the situation but Zibrak had not been notified. But no one had thought Yost and Palmer *were* in critical condition the nurse reported. No one had expected them to die.

It was approaching eleven by the time the patient from the psychiatric ward was calm enough to be returned to the floor where he belonged. Now Zibrak was free to respond to the call from 5East, but before he could do this his pager sounded once again. A patient was arresting in the CCU. When Zibrak arrived, the surgery intern on duty that night was already in the unit attending to the arresting patient.

At not much past eleven-thirty, while the two were still engaged in the CCU, another Code sounded. The new emergency was on 5West. Leaving the surgery intern to finish the resuscitation, Zibrak ran to the fifth floor where another patient had been found without a pulse, unresponsive, and not breathing. This was Alex Brock, a nurse told him. She had found him this way, pulse weak, lips gray.

Zibrak began cardiac massage, pressing down hard on Brock's chest. Mike McLeod, the surgery intern, arrived a few minutes later and started intubation, but he found that Brock's vocal cords were swollen. The tube could not slip between them. McLeod and Zibrak took turns trying to force the tube into place without success. And then, as they struggled, they heard a nurse call, "There's another one in here across the hall." McLeod stayed with Brock. Zibrak ran to the new emergency.

When he entered the room, he saw that the patient in trouble was Douglas Berry, a man whom he had visited daily since Berry's admission to the hospital. Berry was being treated for what had been diagnosed as an infected hip joint. Now he lay staring at the ceiling. He had no pulse.

Frantically Zibrak began cardiac massage, but Berry's heart failed to respond to the compression. Turning, Zibrak called to a nurse to bring him the equipment he needed to administer an electric shock to the heart. This was a small device with two metal paddles. Zibrak placed the paddles on Berry's chest on either side of his heart. Then pressing a switch, he activated a mild electric current that, running between the paddles, would travel directly through the heart, hopefully restoring its movement. That didn't happen. Twice Zibrak tried the procedure but could find no evidence that Berry's heart was responding. He called for epinephrine. It was only then, after he had injected the drug directly into the heart, that there was movement, a pulse, a return to life.

Across the hall McLeod was not having comparable success. Abandoning his efforts to make Brock's throat accept an intubation tube, he and another surgery resident had together performed a tracheostomy, creating a small hole in Brock's trachea through which they could insert a tube that would permit air to enter Brock's lungs, bypassing his swollen vocal cords. But this was not enough.

Alex Brock died shortly after midnight. Douglas Berry died ten days later, having never regained the brain function that lack of oxygen had destroyed.

CHAPTER 7

Early on the afternoon on Friday, the fifteenth of August, the head nurse in the ICU received a telephone call from Dr. Bishop. He needed a bed in the ICU for a patient just admitted to the medical service. There were no beds available, she told him. The unit was full. Bishop suggested that they might transfer a patient out of the ICU onto one of the surgery wards, saying he would call Dr. Freier's office to inquire about this possibility.

Shortly after four o'clock Bishop went to the ICU, intending to meet Freier there to discuss a transfer. While he waited for Freier to arrive, he stood talking to the head nurse on the three-thirty to midnight shift about which patient might be moved.

Around them the unit buzzed with activity. Teams of residents and students from both the medical and surgical services were making rounds. The nursing shifts were in the process of changing, those going off duty hurrying to finish their work while others were gathered in a room just off the unit, briefing the new shift on the condition of the patients.

Bishop and the head nurse stood not far from the door to the isolation room where Arthur Lenz lay. Lenz was a patient that Bishop felt might be transferred. His condition seemed to have become stable enough to warrant such a move. But now, as they stood together discussing this possibility, a nurse appeared in the doorway of Lenz's room and called out, "Mr. Lenz isn't breathing."

At that moment Anne Hill was in her office, giving two medical students a tutorial. She remembered hearing the phone in her outer office being lifted and banged down, then lifted again. Knowing her secretary had left for the day, she called, "Who's that? What are you doing?" It was an anesthesia resident, who replied. "There's an arrest in the ICU. I was calling to see if they need me."

Hill jumped up. "You don't *call* to ask if you're needed!," she cried. "You go!" And then, telling him to bring her resuscitation box, she headed for the ICU.

Dr. Lucy Goodenday, the head of the Cardiology Section, was on the eighth floor in the middle of a phone conversation when her pager began sounding an alert. There could be a cardiac problem, she thought, and she might be needed. Terminating the conversation, she hurried to respond.

By the time she arrived on the third floor the resuscitation was well under way, Weber and McLeod at work. She stood with Bishop and Hill outside Lenz's room and together they watched the procedure. In a short time Freier joined them. This may have been the first of the unexplained arrests to be witnessed by members of the senior staff, but it would not be the last that afternoon.

After a few minutes, observing outside Lenz's room, Dr. Goodenday could see that she wasn't needed. Lenz's heart was not a problem. And so she started toward the CCU, thinking she would check on patients there.

A group of doctors was standing just outside the door to the unit. She approached them, meaning to stop and talk, but as she neared the door, she glanced into the room and saw a patient who appeared to be agitated.

This was a patient she knew. She had seen him in consultation. He was Jordan Olson, the forty-nine-year-old owner of an auto body shop in a small town in western Michigan. He was being monitored for a heart condition and was scheduled for open heart surgery at University Hospital the following week. Goodenday remembered him as a cheerful man, but this afternoon he appeared apprehensive. She decided to check.

As she approached she saw that a nurse was standing at his bedside. It appeared to her that Olson was trying to speak to the nurse, but somehow couldn't. Taking a quick look at the cardiac monitor beside his bed and seeing no indication of a problem with his heart, she drew closer and began to ask him questions.

Was he having chest pain? she asked him. Olson shook his head. Was he choking? Again, a head shake. Well, was he having trouble breathing, she asked, because it looked to her as if he was. This time he nodded.

At first Goodenday wondered whether it might be anxiety causing the problem, anxiety in response to the excitement in the ICU. She asked him to take a few slow, deep breaths, but his next breath was extremely shallow. And then, as she watched, he stopped breathing entirely.

Quickly Goodenday turned to the nurse and told her to bring an airway and an ambu-bag at once. She was prepared to begin mouth-to-mouth resuscitation while she waited for the equipment, but as she leaned over Olson, ready to begin this procedure, she realized that the nurse hadn't moved. She was simply standing there as if she hadn't understood the order. "This is a respiratory arrest!," Goodenday cried. "Get me what I need immediately!" And then she turned and called into the corridor for help. Almost before she turned back to Olson, people were rushing into the room.

Anne Hill remembered hearing the call as she stood outside Lenz's room, ready to offer assistance if it were needed. Hearing Goodenday's voice, she turned at once and ran to the CCU. There, she remembered, a nurse or respiratory therapist was already ambu-bagging Olson but not doing an adequate job of it, she thought. Olson was blue. "And I couldn't see much movement in his chest. So, shoving the other aside, I took over the ambu-bag myself and asked for intubation equipment. But I knew I had to be careful," she said. "I didn't know this patient's history."

As Hill explained it, inserting a laryngoscope into a patient's throat will stimulate the vagus nerve, which lies in that region. This stimulation can cause a slowing of the heart rate and, in Olson's case, because his heart was the problem, this slowing could be dangerous for him. She had to proceed with caution.

"I asked the nurse in the doorway to get me some 4 percent lidocaine," she said. (Lidocaine is a local anesthetic in liquid form, which, when sprayed into the throat, will relax the vocal cords and calm the vagus nerve.) "She came back with 2 percent. I told her I wanted 4 percent. She told me there was no such thing. Well, I was more than annoyed. I said, 'Don't you dare say that to me! There's 4 percent on the cart out there. Get it now!' So off she went again."

While Hill waited for the lidocaine, she continued to ventilate Olson with the ambu-bag, speaking to him quietly, explaining what she was going to do, and telling him that everything would be all right. When the nurse returned with the proper anesthetic, Hill asked to have a syringe filled, and then she sprayed the liquid into Olson's throat. A few minutes later she began the intubation. Dr. Goodenday stood nearby, monitoring Olson's heart rhythm.

When, at length, the intubation was complete, the ventilator pumping and Olson's heart stabilized, the doctors had time to speak to one another. Hill asked whether Goodenday had witnessed Olson's arrest from the start. Goodenday said that she had. "Well, what did it look like?," Hill asked.

Surprising herself, Goodenday replied, "To me it looked like curare."

CHAPTER 8

Curare is a substance derived from certain plants growing in the jungles of South America. Indians in the rain forests of the Amazon are known to poison the tips of their arrows with the substance for use in hunting. Curare will quickly paralyze any animal pierced by an arrow so treated.

Medically, the word refers to a class of drugs that disrupt communication between nerve endings and muscle receptors, leaving the muscles paralyzed. These are synthetic curares, used only in highly controlled situations, as in the operating room, where their paralyzing effects on the diaphragm can be compensated for with mechanical ventilation.

The drugs are not an anesthetic. They do not obliterate pain but are used in conjunction with anesthesia to facilitate the surgery. In an abdominal operation, for example, the drug will immobilize the abdominal muscles, permitting the surgeon to enter the area, perform the surgery, and close the wound without tension or resistance from the surrounding muscles. When the surgery is complete, the effects of the drug can be reversed with an antidote.

Pancuronium bromide is one of this class of curare-type drugs. It is a nondepolarizing muscle relaxantgenerally known by its trade name Pavulon.

Pavulon was kept stocked in the operating rooms. It was stocked in the ICU as well and, of course, in the Pharmacy. When Goodenday mentioned curare, Hill must have thought about Pavulon and its availability. But there were other muscle relaxants used and stocked in the hospital. One of these was succinylcholine, the drug that, almost a month earlier, Hill had suspected as a possible cause of the shaking observed when Leonard Meadows's arrest began.

But there had been no shaking in Jerrold McDougal's case. Goodenday said she had observed none. It was unlikely then, that if McDougal had been injected with a muscle relaxant it had been succinylcholine.

It was just then, as Hill was pondering the problem, that Bishop and Freier entered the CCU and Freier, doubtless also remembering Meadows's case, reported that shaking had not been a part of Lenz's arrest either. Hill recalled the next moment as one of inspiration. "I said to them, 'Well, I'm going to get a peripheral nerve stimulator and test these patients.' So I called the operating room and asked to have a nerve stimulator and four needles brought down at once."

A peripheral nerve stimulator is a device that Hill used routinely in the operating room as a means of determining the level of muscle relaxant in a patient's body during surgery. In this way she could control the level of the drug, raising it, if needed, as the surgery progressed.

Inserting two needles into the patient's inner arm along the ulnar nerve, she would attach wires projecting from the handheld stimulator to the needles. Through the wires she could send an electric current from the stimulator into the ulnar nerve.

Typically, as the current artificially reestablished the connection between nerve and muscle, the patient's fingers would begin to twitch. In a patient who had received a nondepolarizing drug, the twitches exhibited a characteristic pattern.

A doctor with Anne Hill's training and experience could quickly recognize the pattern and identify the drug and its level in the patient's body. "I had done it so often," she said. "If it was Pavulon causing the arrests, the nerve stimulator would indicate that."

So now, with the stimulator in hand, she went to test Lenz. He was lying motionless, a mechanical ventilator pumping air into his lungs, but Hill suspected that if he was suffering the effects of a muscle relaxant he was aware of what was going on around him. The drug would not have rendered him unconscious. He would hear her if she spoke to him.

And so she asked him to open his eyes. There was no response. She asked him to squeeze her hand. She asked him to lift his head. Lenz could not respond to any of these requests. "And so I took his arm," Hill said. "I cleansed the skin and inserted the needles along the ulnar nerve. I connected the stimulation wires. I switched on the current." Lenz's fingers twitched.

As the stimulator continued to supply current, Hill took Lenz's hand and felt his palm for the characteristic pattern of twitches. Then she nodded. The pattern was there. For Hill this was evidence that Lenz had certainly received a nondepolarizing muscle relaxant. "There was nothing else that could produce this picture," she said.

It was time to test Olson.

Returning to the CCU, she repeated the procedure, inserting the needles, connecting the wires. When she switched on the current, the results were exactly as they had been with Lenz. McDougal's fingers began to twitch, and Hill could feel the pattern in his palm.

"That's when I decided I was going to reverse these patients," she said. "I was going to give them the antidote we use in the OR [operating room]." Their response to the antidote would provide positive proof of the presence of a muscle relaxant.

"I hoped I was wrong," Hill said. If the antidote was effective it would mean that both patients had received a drug not ordered for them, not recorded in their charts, and given, it seemed, through their intravenous apparatus solely for the purpose of poisoning them. "But it was the only thing to do," she said.

Hill sent a medical student to the operating room to bring back an unopened bottle of the antidote, neostigmine, and an unopened bottle of atropine, which was meant to counteract any slowing of the patients' hearts as a result of the neostigmine. Because Lenz's was the stronger heart, she decided to begin the procedure with him.

While Freier, Bishop, and Goodenday watched, she opened the two bottles and asked to have syringes filled. She repeated the nerve stimulator test once again, obtaining the same results. Again she asked Lenz to open his eyes, to squeeze her hand, and he could do neither. Hill paused a moment, then asked for the syringes.

Taking the syringe filled with atropine, she injected the drug into the IV bag hanging from the rack beside Lenz's bed. Next she injected the neostigmine, then turned up the IV monitor to accelerate the speed of the drip. She waited. Then once more she asked Lenz to open his eyes. "And within two minutes he started to raise his eyebrows," she said. "Within ten minutes he squeezed my hand so hard it hurt."

She returned to Olson's bedside. Freier, Bishop, and Goodenday watched as she repeated the injection of the antidote, watched as Olson began to move and blink.

If these doctors had had any remaining doubts about the presence of a muscle relaxant in the patients' bodies, the effect of the antidote must have erased them. This was proof of cause at last. But it was proof that led to an inescapable conclusion. Somewhere in the hospital someone was deliberately attacking patients, someone with access to Pavulon and the medical knowledge to use it, someone who could move through the hospital floor to floor and bed to bed without causing the least suspicion.

The doctors stood in silence beside Olson's bed. The idea that there was someone in the hospital purposely injecting patients with a potentially lethal drug seemed inconceivable, too terrible to contemplate. Yet the events of the past hour made such a possibility difficult to deny.

As they stood without speaking, a nurse appeared in the doorway. A third patient had arrested while the doctors were busy with Olson.

This third patient was Robert Lippy, the ex-Marine being treated for a gunshot wound. In an isolation room not far from the room where Olson lay, Lippy had been found limp, blue, and not breathing.

When the doctors reached Lippy, a mechanical ventilator was breathing for him, but, like the others, he lay motionless. Hill set about testing him with the nerve stimulator, injecting the needles and attaching the wires, but in a few minutes she was able to judge from the results she was obtaining that Lippy had received the paralyzing dose too recently to be ready for the antidote. As Hill explained later, "You can't give, say, six milligrams of Pavulon, then reverse it five minutes later. You have to let it wear off a bit. I could tell from the nerve stimulator that he wasn't in a fit state to be reversed."

This meant that very recently someone had entered Lippy's isolation room intending to inject the muscle relaxant. While the doctors were gathered only steps away, someone had entered, injected the drug, and left the room unnoticed. Was this, then, a person so familiar in the unit that he or she could come and go without attracting any particular attention? It seemed so. How else to explain this third attack? The doctors were appalled.

When she judged that sufficient time had passed to allow a weakening of the drug in Lippy's body, Hill returned to his room and administered the nerve stimulator test again. This time the nerve stimulator indicated he was ready for the antidote. Hill injected the neostigmine. In minutes Lippy opened his eyes. Soon he was able to squeeze her hand.

Hill was stunned and shaken. When she felt she could leave the ICU, she returned to her office, wanting to be alone with her thoughts. "I sat," she said, "and I thought. I knew murder had been attempted. I didn't know by whom, but I believed that everyone in the hospital was under suspicion. And I thought that by now whoever it was would know that I knew what it was they had done."

CHAPTER 9

That afternoon when the others left Olson's room to attend to Lippy, Dr. Goodenday stayed behind. She knew that McDougal could not speak because of the breathing apparatus in his mouth and throat, but she thought he might nod or shake his head if she were to ask him a question. Standing at his bedside she asked him whether he had received any medications in the vein just before his arrest occurred, explaining that by "in the vein" she meant through his IV tubing.

Olson seemed to understand. He became animated. He nodded.

Goodenday looked at the chart beside his bed, checking for any authorized medication that might have been administered close to the time of the arrest and found nothing recorded. Was he positive? She asked him. Could he be remembering a later injection, one given to him by Dr. Hill when she administered the antidote? Olson shook his head. Gesturing with his hands, he indicated the intravenous bag on the rack beside him.

Dropping them, he pantomimed his sudden loss of power to move or speak.

Dr. Goodenday hesitated. Did he know who had given him this injection?, she asked. Olson nodded. Could he write the name if he knew it? Another nod. And then, taking the paper and pen she offered, Olson began to write.

The name slanted on the page, printed in large, shaky block letters: "PIA."

This was not a name Dr. Goodenday recognized. She had no idea to whom it might belong. But she was determined to safeguard the paper. If there was a killer in the hospital, one whom Olson could identify, then the printed name on the page could put him in danger. Taking the paper from him, signing and dating it, she left the room and went into the ICU to find Bishop. She asked him to lock the paper away.

By evening Bishop's office on the fifth floor had become a sort of command center, as he said. A locked drawer in his desk was serving as a repository for evidence. In addition to Olson's note there were the IV bags that Anne Hill had ordered removed from the arresting patients' racks and labeled as evidence. She had ordered urine specimens collected and labeled as well, and these she hand delivered to Bishop's office. If murder were the reality, such evidence would be vitally important. Now both the bags and the specimens lay in the locked drawer, waiting to be taken to a laboratory to be analyzed for the presence of Pavulon.

Arriving in Bishop's office shortly before seven to deliver the specimens, Hill had found him pondering the death of a patient on the fifth floor late that afternoon. The patient had suffered an unexplained arrest, he told her. And there was another on the fifth floor who had arrested at about five-thirty, possibly close to the time of the other's death. To him these looked like Pavulon arrests he said. He asked Hill to test the surviving patient.

When she walked into Sheldon Rose's four-bed room she saw a small, white-haired man pulling at his sheets. There seemed to be little point in testing him, she thought. If he could make voluntary movements with his arms, it indicated that in the time that had passed since his arrest the effects of the drug, if present, had had time to wear off. Nevertheless, she tested him, and, although she found no evidence of the drug, she was unwilling to say that it had not been present earlier.

Five arrests in two hours. Three of them certainly caused by Pavulon injections. The two others highly suspicious. Hill was deeply troubled. She returned to the ICU to make notes in the charts of the patients who had arrested there, not having had time to do it earlier. Now she sat, painstakingly recording the testing she had done and the antidotes she had administered. She was tired. The events of the day weighed on her heavily. She was ready to go home, but she was apprehensive. It was approaching nine o'clock. Her car was in a parking lot behind the hospital. It was a lonely walk in the dark.

"I was scared," she said. "I was afraid that whoever had done these things would try to harm me to stop me telling what I knew. My husband was out of town. I couldn't call him to come for me. I had to get home on my own.

When she entered the hospital lobby, the security guard, usually seated there, was nowhere in sight. For a moment she hesitated. "Then I saw a man coming in the front door. He was a nice-looking man. I went up to him and said, 'Would you mind standing here at the door a few minutes? I am going to the parking lot. If you don't see a blue Fiat Spider drive out in five minutes, will you call the police and send them to the parking lot for me?"

Hill was not alone in her anxiety. All those who had witnessed the testing and the effects of the antidotes were anxious. The hospital had become a frightening place. The responsibility for patient safety was immense. If, in fact, a killer was roaming the building, attacking for no apparent reason, many patients could be at risk. Action had to be taken.

That evening Freier joined Bishop in the latter's office, shattered by Hill's discovery. They agreed that immediate measures were needed. Precautions must be put in place, the authorities called in, and an investigation begun at once. Because the hospital was federal property, this would mean calling the Federal Bureau of Investigation (FBI). Arnold Mouish, the hospital director, was the person to initiate that action, but they had not been able to reach him even though they had called repeatedly since late afternoon.

Now, failing to reach him once again, they decided they could wait no longer. Freier put in a call to Robert Dawson, the assistant director, and explained the situation. Dawson appeared in Bishop's office almost at once, and together the three men began to plan a course of action.

They called the hospital pharmacist, asking him to come to collect the urine specimens and IV bags to be taken to the University Hospital laboratory for testing. They ordered the stock of IV bags in storage checked for any evidence of tampering. They called the chief of nursing, Gloria Nunley, and asked her to come to Bishop's office to answer questions and perhaps identify the individual named in Olson's note. At about nine o'clock they finally reached Mouish.

Mouish had been away on leave since the first of August. Returning only earlier that day, he was unaware of the arrests that had occurred in his absence and was appalled to hear what Freier and Bishop had to say. He would be there immediately, he said.

Having arrived at Bishop's office, Mouish asked Nunley to compile a list of the arrests with dates and times and to identify the nursing personnel on duty at those times in an effort to establish any patterns that might be meaningful. Late as it was, he and Freier telephoned Chicago to speak to the supplier of the IV solutions used in the hospital. They managed to reach a representative of the company, who assured them that no other hospital the company supplied had reported anything like what they were describing. And wouldn't it be unlikely, he asked, that if contaminated solutions *were* being distributed they would all find their way to Ann Arbor?

Mouish and Freier conceded that it *would* be unlikely. Nevertheless, at that moment patients throughout the hospital were receiving IV solutions from these bags and the men were taking no chances. They ordered all bags confiscated. Until contamination could be ruled out in the laboratory they would replace them with bags obtained from other hospitals in the area where similar problems were not occurring

Contamination, if it existed, was an extremely serious problem, but it might have been an easier one to accept than the frightening alternative facing the group in Bishop's office that night. Deliberate acts? Attempted murder?

At 10:00 p.m. Mouish called the FBI office in Detroit.

CHAPTER 10

Shortly after ten o'clock that night a ringing telephone roused Gary Calhoun from his bed. Calhoun, assistant to the chief of the medical service, was half asleep when he picked up the phone and recognized Bob Dawson's voice. With growing incredulity he listened as Dawson described the situation and recounted the events of the afternoon. Mouish had called in the FBI, Dawson told him. A local agent was expected at the hospital that night. "I told him I'd be right in," Calhoun said. By the time he reached the hospital, the agent, Eugene Ward, was there, speaking with Mouish, Freier, and Bishop.

Evidently Ward had already heard enough to think it was possible that a crime or crimes had been committed. Not long after Calhoun arrived in Bishop's office, Ward put in a call to Richard Delonis, head of criminal prosecutions in the US Attorney's Office in Detroit. The two agreed that an investigation should begin at once.

Logically the ICU was the place to begin. As Mouish reported later, "We felt it was essential to immediately conduct professional, in-depth interviews with personnel assigned to the ICU as they came off duty at midnight." These were the nurses and aides who had been in the unit when the arrests were occurring. Among them was a nurse known as Pia or P.I.

It was past eleven when Calhoun and Ward walked into the small, empty office that would serve as headquarters for the interviews. Nursing shifts in the ICU were changing. Calhoun hurried to summon those preparing to go off duty.

In a statement prepared for the FBI some four months later, Calhoun documented the interviews that took place that night, using notes he had taken at the time.

Ward interviewed two nurses' aides and two RNs, Calhoun recalled, beginning with the assistants, asking them to describe their activities and whereabouts as the arrests were occurring. Both described going about their routine duties, taking temperatures and blood pressure readings, attending to patients' various needs. In response to Ward's question, both denied seeing anyone in the unit who was a stranger to them or had no good reason to be there.

Third to be interviewed was Leonora Perez, a slender, dark-haired RN, a native of the Philippines. Calhoun remembered Ward's questions to her as being much the same ones he had asked the aides. She, too, had been attending patients, she said, dispensing medications. When Mr. Lenz's arrest began she had been standing near his room. Earlier she had given him his medications but no injection. She thought she had given no patient an injection that day.

It is not clear how long each of these interviews lasted or at what time the last one began. In any case it was very late when Ward began to speak with Filipina Narciso.

Calhoun stated in his report, "We knew at the time of this interview that Miss Narciso was the nurse identified by Mr. Olson as having given him a shot just a few seconds before he blacked out in respiratory arrest." They knew this because earlier, in Bishop's office, Gloria Nunley had recognized the nickname Pia as belonging to Narciso.

Now she sat before Ward, another young RN from the Philippines. She was small, slightly plump, and seemingly uncertain. Her dark hair was cut in a sensible bob. Her smile was shy. Her voice was quiet. Sitting with her hands folded in her lap, she spoke politely, answering Ward's questions.

She had been speaking with Dr. Bishop, standing near the door to Mr. Lenz's isolation room when the arrests began, she said. Suddenly Mr. Lenz yelled and gave signs that he could not breathe. She went into the room. Both she and Leonie Perez had gone into the room to stay and help with the resuscitation.

Then, while still in Mr. Lenz's room, she had learned that a patient in the CCU was in trouble, so she left Mr. Lenz to go there. This was Mr. Olson. He was upset by the increased activity in the ICU she said. His heart monitor was indicating missed beats. He complained that his IV tubing was too short and hurting him. To make him more comfortable she had added extension tubing to his IV line. Then she returned to Mr. Lenz's room.

Did Mr. Olson know her as Pia? Ward asked. She nodded. Had she explained what she was doing when she added the extension tubing? She had. Finally Ward asked how much prior to the beginning of his arrest she had added the extra tubing. Possibly twenty or thirty minutes earlier, she said.

To Ward, Narciso must have seemed an unlikely suspect in spite of Olson's identification. Olson's note, after all, had been scrawled by a man who had undergone a frightening and perhaps disorienting experience, one that might have left him confused. It is easy to understand Ward doubting that this small, courteous young woman, sitting so patiently answering his questions, could be responsible for a ghastly series of poisonings and murders.

CHAPTER 11

While Ward conducted interviews, the group in Bishop's office continued to discuss the situation facing them. Any hope that the arrests had been the result of accident or error was no longer tenable. Trust, which is indispensable to the day-to-day functioning of any hospital, had become a casualty, replaced in one short afternoon by suspicion and fear. In its absence, much would have to change.

Security in the hospital had never been stringent. Visitors came and went freely in the building. Volunteers, maintenance workers, and clerical and support staff moved freely, too, none wearing the sort of identification badge now required in most hospitals. Many medications were easily accessible in unlocked storage. Pavulon was stocked in an unlocked refrigerator in the ICU as well as in the operating rooms.

On the night of the fifteenth the doctors in Bishop's office ordered Pavulon and other muscle relaxants secured under lock and key as narcotics always had been. They discussed clustering those patients who had IVs running in a central location where they could be closely watched. They agreed to assign additional nurses to the ICU and ordered that any nurse giving a patient an injection was to do this from then on in the presence of a witness.

Staff coming on duty the morning of the sixteenth entered a hospital that was acknowledging a crisis.

That same morning Mouish called the VA Central Office in Washington to report on the situation. At about eleven o'clock Ward and Calhoun went to the CCU to see Olson.

Olson was as Dr. Goodenday had left him, intubated and unable to speak. "But he could move," Calhoun recalled. "He could write." When Ward handed him paper and a ballpoint pen and asked him to write the name of the person who had given him the injection just prior to his arrest, Olson again wrote the name, PIA. Could he describe this individual? Ward asked. Olson nodded. Slowly he wrote 'Mexican looking.' And could he recall anything this individual might have been holding? Ward asked. "He drew a syringe," Calhoun reported. "There was no mistake it was a picture of a syringe with a needle."

Yet, despite Olson's apparent certainly, Ward seemed to have remaining doubts. Once more that weekend he and Calhoun went to the CCU to see the patient. Ward had a plan. He proposed bringing Filipina Narciso and two or three other ICU nurses into Mr. Olson's room, one nurse at a time. Under the pretext of needing information, he would ask each to demonstrate how she would add extension tubing to Olson's IV line should that be necessary. His objective was to determine whether or not Olson could make a positive identification, choosing Narciso from among the others.

He explained the plan to Olson who, extubated and able to speak now, agreed to cooperate and make no identification until each nurse had left the room. This settled, Ward and Calhoun went into the ICU to summon nurses.

"There were other Asian nurses working in the ICU who might fit Mr. Olson's description of 'Mexican looking,'" Calhoun wrote in his report. "We came back into the room with Leonora Perez." (Perez, of course, was also from the Philippines and might be thought to resemble Narciso.) "We asked her to point out where an extension tubing would be hooked on," Calhoun reported. "She did this and then she left the room." But she was not Pia. Olson shook his head.

They repeated the experiment with a second nurse. Again Olson shook his head and said that she was not the one. Then they brought in Narciso. "As soon as she walked into the room Mr. Olson's cardiac monitor began to emit erratic beeps," Calhoun recalled. "This person really upset him." And when she left the room Olson made clear that she was the nurse who had given him the injection. "Yes," Olson said, "Yes."

"It appeared to me at that time that there was no question in Mr. Olson's mind that Miss Narciso was the nurse he remembered," Calhoun said. But on Monday he began to hear rumors in the hospital that Olson was claiming it had been a man who had given him the injection.

Once again Ward and Calhoun went to the CCU, this time accompanied by Mark Gullickson, assistant to Mouish. Ward asked Olson about the rumor. Olson denied it entirely. He had not changed his story. He remembered the arrest in detail. He had just awakened from a nap, he said. The nurse, Pia, came over to his bed. As she approached he saw that she was carrying a small piece of tubing and a syringe. She told him that she was going to put an extension on his IV tubing so that the solution could run more freely. Then, with the syringe, she injected something into the tubing. She injected it very rapidly, then turned and walked away. He began to feel a burning sensation in his arm. He thought he must have been given the wrong medication. He tried to call out and couldn't speak. He couldn't move or open his eyes, and then he couldn't breathe. He remembered it all very clearly.

When Ward asked whether anyone had tried to get him to change his story, Olson recalled a nurse who had. She kept asking him if he wasn't mistaken about what he remembered, he said. But he had no intention of changing his mind. It had been exactly as he reported.

Earlier that day Ward, together with Calhoun and Gullickson, had interviewed Robert Lippy, the last patient Anne Hill had injected with neostigmine on the fifteenth. He remembered being groggy, having just awakened from a nap, when he felt someone jiggling the IV in his arm and causing him pain. He turned to look and saw a man with curly, dark brown hair just leaving the room. He judged the man to be five foot ten or eleven in height and wearing a green surgical shirt. He saw this man, and then he collapsed.

A third patient interviewed that day could remember little of his arrest. He had been very, very sleepy, he said. There had been someone in the room, he thought, someone at the foot of his bed, but that was all he could recall.

Clearly Olson's account was the most comprehensive and involved the most possibly useful information. But what to make of the man with the curly, dark brown hair or a tall man in a green shirt who had been observed by a patient's visitors running out of the ICU as a Code 7 light began to flash?

CHAPTER 12

Between July 1 and August 15 there had been fifty-one arrests in the hospital involving thirty-six patients, several of whom had arrested more than once. Yet it was far from clear how many of these arrests could be attributed to deliberate acts. Hospital records covering a comparable period the preceding year registered only twelve arrests, a number compatible with statistics indicating that eight a month or two per week was the norm. Fifty-one arrests left thirty-nine outside the norm.

A list including only those arrests that appeared definitely suspicious was what the FBI needed to proceed with its investigation. Two committees set about supplying such lists.

An in-house review began at once. The weekend following Anne Hill's testing Drs. Freier and Bishop and other physicians on the VA staff began examining patients' charts again, trying to identify arrests that appeared particularly suspicious. On Monday, the eighteenth, a second committee was assembled comprised of physicians from the University of Michigan Medical School and the School of Public Health.

Headed by Dr. Jeoffrey Stross from the Department of Postgraduate Medicine at the Medical School, this committee set out on a parallel quest. In consultation with the VA doctors who had attended the arresting patients and with physicians from the Centers for Disease Control, the committee began an evaluation of patient records, seeking to assess each arrest for a natural or suspicious cause.

Dr. Stross described this as an epidemiologic investigation, explaining that the committee approached the situation as it would an epidemic, looking at factors of time and place, persons affected, the agent or cause of the problem, and the way or ways in which the agent was transmitted.

The committee began by assigning the arrests to groups labeled "no suspicion," "moderate suspicion," and "high suspicion." Arrests judged nonsuspicious were ones that could be attributed to the patient's disease process and condition. They had not been unexpected. In contrast, arrests labeled highly suspicious *were* unexpected and had occurred in patients whose condition had seemed satisfactory. Among these arrests there was no evidence of cardiac involvement. The resuscitations had been unusually successful even though the patients had remained flaccid, or unmoving, for some time following the arrests. Many seemed never to have lost consciousness.

As Anne Hill had recognized, these were effects compatible with the presence of a muscle-paralyzing agent, but it was not clear that all highly suspicious arrests had been caused by the same agent or that the agent had been administered in the same manner. Although it seemed probable that this was the case, further study and analysis would be needed before such a conclusion could be substantiated.

In its investigation the committee determined that most of the highly suspicious arrests had occurred between 4:00 p.m. and midnight, a great many concentrated in the ICU. When such arrests occurred elsewhere in the hospital, they often followed a slightly earlier low-suspicion arrest and took place nearby, in an adjoining room or across a hall. All patients in the high-suspicion group had been receiving IV fluids, and almost all had had a Volutrol apparatus attached to the IV line. This is a device that permits an individual to inject a patient with a substance and leave the vicinity before the effects of the injection begin to be felt.

An epidemiologic investigation seeks to identify those factors contributing to the spread of an epidemic. When the factors are controlled or removed, the spread of the epidemic is expected to abate. The epidemic of VA arrests did just that. Once muscle relaxants were placed in locked storage and patients receiving IV fluids were segregated on a special ward under tight security, the unexplained arrests ceased. There had been none since late afternoon on the fifteenth.

The weekend following August 15 local FBI agents had begun setting up a headquarters on the hospital's fifth floor. Rooms formerly occupied by patients became offices where files, hospital records, and data collected from the medical investigating committees would soon begin to accumulate. Other rooms were reserved for the interviews about to take place.

The FBI's plan was to interview all those hospital employees who came in contact with patients and might be able to provide useful information concerning the arrests. In a hospital the size of the Ann Arbor VA, the scope of such an undertaking was immense. The hospital employed nearly eight hundred people—medical staff, nursing staff, and support and maintenance personnel—any one of whom might have seen or heard something that could be relevant to the investigation. Besides interviews with employees, agents intended to speak with all the affected patients and their visitors. Within two weeks of the fifteenth of August there were twenty agents in the hospital, working in a strictly cordoned-off wing on the fifth floor.

CHAPTER 13

On the morning of August 18, Arnold Mouish had telephoned Dr. John Chase, the chief medical director at the VA Central Office, asking him to send a team of experts from the Central Office to assist in the effort under way. On the same morning Dr. Bishop called a meeting of the members of the house staff, intending to inform them about what had happened in the hospital during the preceding three days.

It seems likely that a good many of these young doctors already knew. Several, of course, had been in the ICU when the arrests and reversals were taking place and had been involved in the resuscitations. Yet to hear the chief of the medical service acknowledge the possibility of murder was stunning.

The group stood for several minutes, processing what Bishop had told them. Then a senior resident from the medical service spoke. If patients were being murdered in the hospital, he said, then the house staff should demand that the administration stop all new admissions immediately, accepting only emergency cases, patients in life-or-death situations. There was a rumble of approval. The house staff agreed.

Patients presently in the hospital should be informed of the ongoing investigation, he added. Patients admitted for emergency procedures should be provided with written statements informing them and their families of the situation. A vote was taken. The proposal was approved, and a small group of residents, representing the House Officers' Association, was chosen to take the proposal to Mouish.

Closing the hospital to all but emergency cases was a radical move and one that Mouish was evidently reluctant to consider. But the representatives of the house staff persisted, threatening to take the proposal public if the administration failed to act.

Publicity was what the administration had been hoping to avoid all along, fearing severe damage to the hospital's reputation if news of the arrests became widely known. Closing the hospital to new admissions would surely result in such publicity, but an airing of the house staff's proposal would do the same. Mouish was between a rock and a hard place. That afternoon he took the proposal to a meeting of the senior staff.

Dr. Freier recalled, "That Monday I was in the operating room all day, and I missed the staff meeting. That's when they shut the hospital down. "I was furious. I thought of all the things we should do that wasn't one of them."

Freier was also greatly concerned about the publicity that would follow this action. "That was what I was trying to convince people to avoid, but it happened, and then one of the resident's wives was a reporter on the Ypsilanti paper and, bango!, they just zeroed in."

On Monday afternoon, the eighteenth, the first headline appeared:

"Probe/FBI Studies VA Hospital Death." The words were bannered across the front page of the *Ypsilanti Press*. The accompanying article contained the news: "Arnold Mouish, administrator at the hospital, confirmed today that the VA facility is limiting admissions to emergencies." It went on to report on the situation, saying, "Whether the deaths were accidental, natural or otherwise has not been determined."

Freier remembered, "The publicity just exploded. At this point it just went ballistic."

In fact it was a day or two before the news truly exploded. The *Ypsilanti Press* is a small afternoon daily published in a town neighboring Ann Arbor, chiefly devoted to local news. Its headline was not likely to be much noticed in the wide world of newspaper publishing, but the story *did* make an appearance on the state wire service. Editors at the *Detroit Free Press* picked it up there and sent a reporter to the hospital to check on the situation.

The subsequent article in the August 10 *Free Press* quoted Arnold Mouish as "emphatically denying rumors of foul play," reporting that Mouish claimed the deaths at the hospital involved ill and elderly patients and were not unexpected. But in the same article an FBI agent was quoted as saying, "We are not an agency that does things for the hell of it. We would not be involved unless circumstances indicated it was warranted."

On August 20 a *Free Press* headline asked, "Killer at Large in Veterans' Hospital?" Then the news did begin to explode. That week the disappearance of Teamsters' president Jimmy Hoffa, a story that had occupied front pages for days, began sharing space with reports of the hospital deaths. The media frenzy had begun.

By Tuesday, the nineteenth, the investigative team from the VA Central Office had arrived in Ann Arbor, headed by the deputy chief medical officer, Dr. Laurence Foye. The five-member team made its way into the hospital through groups of reporters. The next day Dr. Foye held a press conference.

It was a hot day. A photograph on the front page of the August 20 *Ann Arbor News* shows Foye, a plump, bespectacled man, mopping his forehead as he stood answering questions. "One of many possibilities is that it was an intentional act," the *News* quotes him saying, apparently referring to only one death, "but so far we have been unable to develop supporting evidence that this was an intentional act."

After listing the drugs under suspicion, Foye said that an analysis of blood and urine specimens being done at the University of Michigan Hospital laboratories was "so far inconclusive." There had been a breakdown in the equipment used for such tests. Repair parts were being flown in and should arrive that afternoon. The tests would continue.

On August 22 the *Ann Arbor News* headline was "Drug Clues Point to VA Murder." Traces of a muscle relaxant had been found in urine specimens in the laboratory, and "The identification of the drug has forced investigators to conclude that recent respiratory arrests at the VA Hospital were murder and attempted murder."

Two days later the *News* quoted Dr. Freier: "We have ruled out completely the possibility of medical coincidence, error, and drug contamination. That leaves us with the fact that some, perhaps many, of the respiratory arrests were caused by someone with intent."

Asked about a possible motivation for the attacks, Freier rejected euthanasia or mercy killing: "The pattern [of respiratory arrests and deaths] is not right. This person is more like an arsonist, starting fires and sitting back to watch what happens."

In the following days, newspaper accounts proliferated across the country and began to appear in many papers abroad. Although there were other big stories that summer, notably the Hoffa disappearance and the kidnapping of Patty Hearst, the Ann Arbor VA deaths seemed to command special interest.

When no new announcements were forthcoming from the hospital administration, reporters found other ways to feed the demand for VA stories. They waylaid families entering and leaving the building, asking for their thoughts about the situation. They questioned any hospital employee who paused long enough to be approached. The administration had prohibited interviews with patients, but an occasional reporter found a way around the prohibition, speaking with a patient who had ventured into one of the public areas.

An *Ann Arbor News* reporter had discovered two such patients drinking coffee in the hospital canteen, identified by the pajamas and robes they were wearing. Presumably they had received the same government memorandum that had been distributed to all patients, informing them of the ongoing investigation, but neither blamed the hospital for what had happened. "I look at it this way," said one, quoted in the August 20 *News*, "everybody makes mistakes. That's why they put erasers on pencils."

Some patients' families were not so ready to exonerate the hospital. The brothers of Roy Custer had hired a lawyer. Custer, who entered the hospital for treatment of a broken hip, had died there four days later following a breathing arrest. His brothers were considering bringing a malpractice suit against the hospital.

And there were other stories. Gregory Wiley, who had died on August 8, was buried before a death certificate was filed, a violation of state law. For an enterprising reporter there was a good deal of information to be gleaned beyond official announcements.

People working in the hospital that summer speak, often with irritation, of the relentless presence of the media, the swarms of reporters in the building, the television trucks parked, almost permanently it seemed, outside. An article in the September 8 *Detroit Free Press* tells of one such irritated young doctor who, stepping off an elevator into the glare of television lights, had a microphone pushed toward him and was asked if he had anything to say. "The doctor took a long look into the camera, paused for a significant moment, and began talking in a slow, solemn voice: 'I would like to say that I will be a candidate for the Presidency in 1976,' he said." Then he handed back the microphone and departed.

Not everyone treated the situation with humor. One physician, who was an intern in the summer of 1975, wrote of the pain he still felt. "That challenging period of training was difficult enough," he wrote, "without mass murder, politics, and a hospital ignoring obviously extraordinary circumstances. It seriously impacted us."

That patients in their care had been murdered can hardly have failed to have an impact on these young doctors. Frustration with the dilatory response of the administration was a recurring theme.

CHAPTER 14

During these weeks routines in the hospital continued as normally as possible. Employees went about their work. But there was a pervasive sense of anxiety in the building. The FBI investigation was entering its third week. Dozens of interviews had taken place, but it seemed that no suspect had been positively identified.

For the FBI, the pressure to identify a suspect or suspects and bring the investigation to a close was intense. That summer the bureau was deeply involved in both the Hoffa case and the Hearst kidnapping and was having little success with either. A third long-running, unsuccessful investigation was not a pleasant prospect.

Agent Dan Russo remembered being in Detroit that summer, at work on the Hoffa investigation, when he was asked to go to Ann Arbor. Russo had some medical knowledge. Most of the agents investigating the arrests had none and were depending on physicians who could interpret the medical terminology for them. "So they kind of wanted me to go out there and say, 'Here's what you should be asking the doctors' or 'Look at the information—see what it adds to the overall investigation,'" Russo said.

When he arrived, the agents on the fifth floor had been working long hours, sifting through the accumulating data. They now had a list provided by the in-house committee of physicians, citing the fifteen arrests considered definitely suspicious. They had a report from Foye's committee about the events on the fifteenth, work schedules for the nursing staff both in the ICU and on the floors, and lists of the medical students, residents, and interns working in the hospital during the six weeks in which the arrests were occurring.

The changeover of the house staff on the first of July, coinciding as closely as it did with the onset of the arrests, seemed possibly significant. Briefly a medical student was under suspicion, but further investigation led nowhere, and no other members of the house staff appear to have been considered suspects.

Interviews with patients were proving disappointing. Most of the patients who had undergone arrests could provide little useful information. Most had been sleeping or only just waking when their arrests began and could remember little or nothing about what had preceded them. Robert Lippy's memory of a man with curly brown hair leaving his room seemed to be heading nowhere. Only Olson's testimony implicating Filipina Narciso appeared to point in a fruitful direction.

Agents interviewed Narciso twice in August, initially on the night of the fifteenth and again on the twenty-sixth. At the second interview she acknowledged that she knew she was a suspect, knew that a patient had named her. But she felt that the medication the patient received following his arrest could have left him disoriented. A day or two later a doctor had told her that the patient, Mr. Olson, had reported that the last person near his bed prior to his arrest had been a man. In fact, she had a note from Olson saying, "It was a man." She spoke of Lippy's memory of a man in a scrub shirt leaving his room as his arrest began. She described the strange behavior of a male medical student in the ICU whom she had had to reprimand for turning off a patient's IV without orders to do so. And besides, she was not known as "Pia," she said, her nickname was "P.I."

Narciso could not have known on the twenty-sixth that within a few days Olson's testimony implicating her in his arrest would change entirely.

A week following his arrest on the fifteenth, Olson had been transferred to University Hospital for open heart surgery. On his return to the VA for recuperation he could no longer recall much of what he had told Ward and Calhoun and contradicted a good deal of what he had said earlier. He no longer remembered the name Pia or the circumstances of the arrest that had been so clear in his mind before his surgery. It was another nurse, he said, who had given him the injection.

Retrograde amnesia, as it is called, is evidently a common, even expected condition following coronary bypass surgery. It is a condition well described in the medical literature. Dr. Stross says that had he known Olson was about to undergo this surgery he would have advised the FBI to tape Olson's testimony before the surgery took place. But this had not been done, and Olson's account was crumbling.

As Agent Russo said, "Now your most damaging evidence isn't there." Laboratories had identified Pavulon in Olson's IV line, and there was the evidence of Anne Hill's drug reversal, "so all of that was built up and, gee, that makes a slam dunk." But without reliable testimony from the FBI's only eyewitness it was far from a slam dunk. Ward's and Calhoun's notes on the interviews with Olson could not be considered hard evidence without Olson's corroboration. His altered account significantly altered the investigation.

CHAPTER 15

2 New Deaths Tied to Breathing Stops

The headline appeared above a story in the *Ann Arbor News* on August 30. Detroit papers carried similar stories, reporting that two patients who had undergone breathing arrests earlier in the month had died on the twenty-seventh. The *News* quoted doctors at the hospital as saying they believed one of the deaths was directly linked to an earlier arrest. No cause had as yet been determined for the second.

On September 1, the *News* reported that Dr. Freier was denying any drug involvement in these deaths. Tests had indicated nothing of this kind, no Pavulon or other muscle relaxant present. But when asked whether the earlier arrests could have weakened the patients' overall condition Freier admitted that this was probable. The papers added these deaths to the total they were reporting.

Early that evening Dr. S. Martin Lindenauer stepped off a plane at the John F. Kennedy International Airport in New York. Lindenauer, the permanent chief of staff at the Ann Arbor VA was returning from a six-month sabbatical in London. The next morning he would fly to Ann Arbor.

Lindenauer, a slender man in his mid-forties, wore the tired expression of a trans-Atlantic passenger. Walking through the doors into the terminal, he saw his brother and sister-in-law among the crowd in the waiting area, and almost at once he knew that something was wrong. His brother's face was somber. Fearing bad news, Lindenauer hurried toward them, asking, "What's happened, Art? What's wrong? Did someone die?" His brother shook his head. "No," he said, "but your hospital nearly has," and handed Lindenauer a sheaf of newspapers.

Lindenauer was stunned. He knew nothing about the situation at the hospital. As he explained it, he and his family had been traveling in Europe for part of July and all of August and would have been difficult to reach. He had seen few newspapers on the trip. But now, as he suddenly realized, he was returning to a crisis.

The next day he entered a hospital shockingly different from the one he'd left six months earlier. He remembered an atmosphere of tension and anxiety. It seemed to him that distrust was lurking in the eyes of everyone he encountered that morning. "And, oh my God, the media," he said. Before he could enter his office, reporters were asking him for statements.

At 7:15 that morning another patient had died, a man who had suffered several earlier arrests. The reporters crowding around Lindenauer wanted him to comment on a mysterious blue liquid that had been found a few days before in the man's IV tubing. Was it some sort of poison? Was it more evidence of attempted murder? By the next day Lindenauer could tell them that the liquid had been tested and was harmless, that it was a cleansing agent used routinely to clear the bladder, but on this first morning back in his office he could hardly have been expected to have answers for all the questions put to him.

In the forefront of his mind that day, and for many days to come, was the survival of the hospital. The restriction of admissions was, he felt, a serious problem. There was a backlog of some forty patients waiting to be admitted for treatment. "It couldn't go on the way it was," Lindenauer said. "If we continued restricting admissions to emergency cases only, we would begin to lose students and medical staff." As he explained it, without a larger patient population at the VA, the university would begin to feel that there were insufficient teaching opportunities for its medical students, interns, and residents and would assign these students and doctors to other hospitals. "In time the VA would cease to exist as a teaching institution," Lindenauer said. He was determined that this should not happen.

On the third of September the hospital announced that admissions would be reopened to nonemergency cases within the next few weeks, bringing the currently limited number of patients to a near-normal census of about 250. New safeguards and added surveillance would accompany the increase, Lindenauer announced, substantially augmenting the safeguards already in place.

Patients receiving IV fluids were to be gathered in a wing on the third floor near the ICU where a security guard stationed in the corridor that ran between these areas could monitor all persons entering either one, staff and visitors alike. Staff would be provided with photo IDs. All visitors would be required to present identification.

On other floors in the hospital, guards would be positioned twenty-four hours a day at the junctions of the corridors between the east and west wings, and anyone wishing to enter would be required to present identification and sign in. Emergency doors leading to stairwells would be fitted with locks permitting exit but not entrance, thus limiting and controlling the passage between floors.

As the new safeguards were put in place, it became clear to all that the hospital administration feared a killer was still at large in the building. Although there had been no unexplained incidents since the fifteenth of August, it seemed that no suspect had yet been identified by the FBI.

In the rumors traveling from floor to floor in the hospital, the word *insane* was common. The killer had to be insane, people said. How else to explain the attacks? Whether the motive was mercy killing, thrill seeking, anger at the administration, or a desire to shut the hospital down, the attacker was clearly psychotic, perhaps someone passed daily in the halls, seen drinking coffee in the canteen, or sharing an elevator between floors, someone insane and dangerous.

CHAPTER 16

The investigation was entering its fourth week when the FBI received the Stross Committee's report assigning levels of suspicion to the group of arrests under scrutiny. Besides classifying these, the report graphically demonstrated that the greatest number of highly suspicious arrests had occurred in the ICU between the hours of four and midnight, helping to confirm the agents' theory that the nursing staff in the unit on the three-thirty to midnight shift was the group most likely to be harboring a suspect.

The report went on to note a clustering phenomenon in the arrests that had occurred on floors outside the ICU. On three occasions an arrest judged to be of low suspicion had been followed within sixty minutes or less by one or two arrests that the committee considered highly suspicious. These subsequent events had occurred in close proximity to the first, in an adjacent room or one across the hall, as if the first emergency had provided an opportunity for the later attacks.

It appeared that members of the ICU nursing staff might be suspects in these cases as well. As Dr. Stross explains, at every cardiopulmonary emergency in the hospital an ICU nurse was *required* to be present, having the experience and skills needed in such an emergency. A Code called for any arrest on any floor would oblige an RN from the ICU to respond at once. It seemed possible, he suggested, that in the rush and confusion of the resuscitation a nurse might slip away long enough to enter an adjoining room or one across the hall.

The agents were well aware that every one of the suspicious arrests that had occurred outside the ICU had taken place in the late afternoon or during the evening, hours that coincided with the three-thirty to midnight nursing shift. Now they learned that at each resuscitation an RN from the unit would have been present as required, and they knew that the RNs on the three-thirty to midnight shift there were most often Filipina Narciso and Leonora Perez. It appeared that a pattern was emerging.

Checking further with nurses and nursing assistants who had been on duty on the fourth and fifth floors while the arrests were taking place, the agents learned that Narciso had been present at a large number of the resuscitations, perhaps most. A nurse on 5West recalled that on August 14, while doctors were struggling with Alex Brock's resuscitation, Narciso had discovered Douglas Berry arresting in a room across the hall. It had been Narciso who called out an alert, and the next day it was Narciso who found Sheldon Rose in distress.

The nursing assistant on 5West remembered that she had seen Narciso approaching from 5East in the late afternoon, carrying a bag of IV solution that she said was needed in the ICU. At the time, the assistant said she wondered why an RN would go on such an errand. It is likely that the agents wondered, too. In the late afternoon on the fifteenth of August all hell was breaking loose in the ICU. It seemed an unlikely time for one of the two RNs in the unit to go looking for an IV bag.

The assistant remembered that she and Narciso had chatted a little, speaking of the number of arrests that day. Then Narciso had walked down the corridor toward the private rooms. A few minutes later she called out that the patient in 510 did not look good. The patient, Sheldon Rose, was arresting.

When Dr. Bishop returned to his office on 5West sometime after five o'clock that afternoon, he found that two patients on the floor had arrested while he was observing the resuscitations in the ICU. One of these patients, Joseph Dyllan, was dead. Sheldon Rose had been successfully resuscitated.

One death and seven arrests in forty-eight hours, four on the fourth and fifth floors. Although the agents had little but circumstantial evidence connecting Filipina Narciso to any of these events, they decided to question her again. On the nineteenth of September she was called for another interview.

Narciso was twenty-nine that summer. Born in Pasay in the Philippines, she had received her nursing degree in Manila, she told the agents. She came from a large Roman Catholic family, and, she explained, it was the practice in her family for the older siblings to find work to finance the education of the younger ones. Her older sister had come to the United States to work as a nurse at the University of Alabama Hospital, helping to pay for Filipina's education. She had urged her sister to come to Alabama after receiving her nursing degree, and Narciso had done that. But in 1972, failing to obtain her nursing license in that state, she had come to the VA in Ann Arbor.

For ten months she had worked on the day shift on 6North. Then she had been assigned to evenings on 4East and later on 5West. From time to time she had worked all over the hospital as a relief supervisor on the evening shift. She knew the building well. In June 1975 she had been assigned to the ICU.

The agents could not have failed to notice the coincidence. Narciso had joined the ICU staff only a month before the arrests began there. But again this was only circumstantial evidence that didn't amount to much. They were investigating thirty-six arrests and five deaths—numbers worthy of a serial killer—while before them sat a small young nurse who was sending money home to help educate her brothers and sisters.

She did not drink alcohol, she said. She was in good health and took no drugs, prescribed or otherwise. This last information surprised the agents, for they knew that in August when Narciso, like other nursing personnel in the ICU, had been asked to take a lie detector test she had refused, claiming that she had taken Valium earlier that day, a drug prescribed for migraine headaches, and she felt she would not do well on the test.

The agents asked about her participation in resuscitations outside the ICU. She agreed that she had responded to a large number, probably more than Leonie Perez. In fact she could remember only two Codes during July and August to which she had *not* responded. But it was her duty, she said.

She spoke of the arrests and resuscitations in the ICU involving Lenz, Olson, and Lippy, saying she had proof of her innocence regarding Olson. Only days after his arrest, Leonie Perez had questioned him, asking about his identification of the nurse who had given him the paralyzing injection. He had written a note, which he gave to Perez. It read, "If I see her again, I will not remember her."

Where *was* the note?, the agents asked.

Perez had given it to her, Narciso said, and she had thrown it away. So it was gone? No, Narciso said, someone had advised her to keep it, and she had done that. She had the note at home.

This was not the first time Narciso had mentioned a note from Olson. The agents reminded her that she had spoken of a note at another interview but claimed the text read "It was a man." Narciso denied this. The only message was the one she had just mentioned, she said.

Several times during the interview Narciso complained that she felt everything pointed to her as responsible for Olson's arrest, but she could not admit to something she had not done. She was innocent, she said. She had nothing to confess.

Narciso, recalling this interview almost a year later, had a very different version to report. The interview had lasted six hours, she told a reporter from the *Ann Arbor News*. There had been two agents questioning her, and they had been harsh. They had yelled at her. "They said, 'You are guilty. You'd better confess because you're guilty and we know you're guilty.'"

According to the article, which appeared in the *Ann Arbor News* on August 29, Narciso remembered one of the agents leaving the room to take a telephone call while the other continued, saying, "You're twenty-nine. If you don't confess your life is all over." "And not only that," Narciso is quoted as saying, "but when he told me my life is over with, he also told me to 'go to church and light a candle—you'll be needing it.'"

A nurse in the ICU remembered Narciso returning from this interview at about eight in the evening, having been with the agents since two that afternoon. She was exhausted, the nurse recalled, nearly collapsing. "They think I'm guilty," was all she said.

That evening the agents telephoned Dr. Lindenauer.

Within a day or two Narciso was transferred from the ICU to the Office of Nursing Education where she would have desk work but no further contact with patients. A spokesman for Dr. Lindenauer, contacted for an article in the *Ann Arbor News*, denied that a nurse (unnamed in the article) had been transferred from the ICU at the prompting of the FBI, adding that the transfer was in no way an indication of guilt.

It seems probable that the transfer did *not* indicate any certainty of guilt. In spite of the suspicions the agents had expressed and the pressure for a confession they apparently exerted, they had too little solid evidence to charge Narciso with murder. It is more likely that the transfer represented the administration's decision to take no chances as long as *any* suspicion existed.

Narciso did not see it that way. To her the transfer was an accusation. She was very upset she told the chief of nursing. She felt she needed legal advice, but she was hesitant. To employ a lawyer in the Philippines was equivalent to an admission of guilt. And she was not guilty. She had done nothing.

CHAPTER 17

Most members of the nursing staff on the three-thirty to midnight shift in the ICU were interviewed more than once as the investigation progressed. Some complained about the frequency and length of the questioning, calling it harassment. It seems probable they knew that as a group they were a focus of suspicion, which could only have increased their discomfort.

Leonora Perez had been questioned several times. As a registered ICU nurse, she, like Narciso, was required to respond to emergencies anywhere in the hospital, and she had been present at a number of the arrests outside the ICU. But, in addition to this, there was the note she had obtained from Olson, the note that Narciso had cited as proof of her innocence. Was Perez the nurse Olson had recalled suggesting to him that his identification of Narciso was a mistake? Was it possible that Perez and Narciso were somehow in league, both involved in the poisonings? The idea may have seemed far-fetched at first, but the agents *did* have some reason to consider the possibility.

In an interview with a nursing assistant working on 4West, they had learned that on the evening of July 30 Perez and Narciso had come onto the floor to visit the patient Chester Rice. They liked visiting patients they had cared for in the ICU once the patients were transferred to other floors, the assistant said. A little earlier they had been on 5West, visiting another patient and his wife. Now they asked if they could visit Rice.

The accounts of what happened next are varied and contradictory. According to a nurse on duty in the ICU that night, Narciso had come running back into the unit shortly after she and Perez left to go visiting. She needed emergency supplies, she said. There was a arrest on 4West.

Later the two nurses told her that when they entered Rice's room they found him on the floor in arrest. Perez had begun closed chest massage. Narciso had run for supplies and to call a Code. This contradicted other testimony the agents had regarding the discovery of Rice's arrest. In that testimony it was a nursing assistant, entering Rice's room to take a blood pressure reading, who had discovered him arresting in his bed. It was Dr. Michael McLeod, responding to her call, who had come into the room to take over.

In later testimony, Perez did not mention finding Rice on the floor. In this account she claimed that Dr. McLeod was already in the room attending to Rice when she and Narciso walked in. While she stayed to help, Narciso ran to call a Code.

But this version of events was questionable, too. If Rice was known to be in arrest when Perez and Narciso came visiting, wouldn't the nursing assistant have told them that? Apparently she hadn't, yet presumably she was the same assistant who had entered his room to take a blood pressure reading. Similarly, if Narciso had run to the ICU for supplies shortly after she and Perez left the unit, how had they had time to pay a visit on 5West first? The stories didn't add up.

In addition there was the testimony of the wife of the patient they had intended to visit on 5West. She remembered that at around nine o'clock that evening she had seen Narciso passing in the corridor outside her husband's room. Narciso had waved to her but had not stopped. She recalled that this was shortly before "a commotion" began in an adjacent room. People came running down the hall, some pushing equipment, she said, and there was a good deal of noise in the next room. Later, after the commotion ended, both Narciso and Perez stopped to speak with her briefly, but she thought Narciso seemed to be in a hurry, saying that they had to go.

Whatever inconsistencies and contradictions exist in these various accounts, some facts are indisputable. Medical records do show that at about nine o'clock on the evening of the thirtieth Howard Jackson arrested in his room on 5West, could not be resuscitated, and was pronounced dead at ten-thirty. Just before ten o'clock Chester Rice arrested on 4West and as this resuscitation was ending a third patient arrested on 4East. During at least some of this time both Perez and Narciso had been observed on the fourth and fifth floors, visiting.

* * *

Like Narciso, Leonora Perez had been born and received her nurse's training in the Philippines. In the early 1970s she had come to the United States to work, employed first at a nursing home in Chicago. In 1972 she had come to Michigan and taken a position at University Hospital on a general surgery floor. In April 1975 she left the university and transferred to the VA because, she said, it provided better benefits and a higher salary. In June 1975 she began work in the ICU, the same month in which Narciso arrived there.

The two had hardly known each other before they began working together in the unit, Perez said. They had no social contact outside the hospital. Unlike Narciso, who was single, Perez was married and the mother of a two-year-old son. When she was not at work she was busy with her family. She and Narciso saw one another only during those hours when both were at work in the unit.

And yet it was Perez who had obtained the note from Olson that seemed to exonerate Narciso. The two apparently made it a practice to visit their former ICU patients together. On the night of the thirtieth of July three patients had arrested on the third and fourth floors while they were visiting, and one of these patients died.

Again this was circumstantial evidence. No one claimed to have seen either Perez or Narciso administering an injection. According to all accounts they were admirable nurses, conscientious and skilled. But the information the agents were compiling was seriously disturbing, and in a short time Perez, too, was reassigned to a position in which she would no longer have responsibility for patient care.

CHAPTER 18

It was nearing the end of September now. Fall was in the air. Behind the hospital the trees had begun to change color, their yellowing leaves a bright contrast to the hospital's dark brick walls.

On 5North, amid clicking keyboards and ringing phones, stacks of files, and mountains of paper, the FBI agents were beginning the sixth week of the investigation. Yet, despite the nearly seven hundred interviews they had conducted and the reams of records they had reviewed, they still had little solid evidence to offer the US prosecutor, Richard Delonis.

The evidence ordinarily produced at a trial for murder—a weapon, an eyewitness, a motive for the act—continued to elude them. And, in fact, had there *been* any murders? There was no certain proof of that either.

Although the doctors who had attended the dying patients reported symptoms that appeared consistent with the presence of a muscle relaxant, these patients had been buried with no tests taken. It was only after Anne Hill's nerve stimulator tests and drug reversals that it became clear such testing might have offered the proof the prosecutor needed.

Laboratory analyses had since identified what appeared to be Pavulon in the urine of two of the patients who had arrested in the ICU on the fifteenth of August. There was good reason to think that the drug would have been found in the urine of earlier arresting patients had it been suspected and tested for. But any such evidence was gone, flushed away.

Pavulon does not remain long in the body. Most will be excreted in the first twenty-four hours following an injection, and all will be gone within a few days. Most patients who survived their arrests that summer would have been clear of the drug days or weeks before Pavulon came under suspicion. But in the case of patients who had died at the time of their arrests, was it possible that Pavulon, unexcreted, might still be harbored in their internal organs?

In consultation with experts at the University of Michigan Hospital and College of Pharmacy, the agents learned that this was indeed a possibility. A well-publicized murder trial on the East Coast had involved just such a circumstance. The body of a woman believed to have been murdered by an injection of a muscle relaxant had been exhumed for testing. Succinylcholine was found in her tissue.

But that was succinylcholine, the agents were warned. Pavulon presented a different problem. Pavulon was a new drug. Although a test existed to identify it in bodily fluids, there was no test yet available to detect it in either living or embalmed human tissue. Such a test would have to be devised in the laboratory, and there was no predicting how long that would take. The agents could be in for a long wait, they were told.

Yet what was the alternative? It was certain that Pavulon had not been ordered for these patients. No such order signed by a physician appeared in any of their charts. If Pavulon could be found in the tissues of their internal organs it would mean that the drug had been injected illicitly with the intention to harm them. It would be evidence of murder. To the prosecutor, and the FBI, exhumations of these patients seemed essential.

And so, shortly after eight-thirty in the morning on the second of October, as early sunlight filtered through the trees at Kalamazoo's Mt. Ever Rest Memorial Park, the grave of Alex Brock was opened on the order of the prosecutor.

Delonis, a sturdy, solidly built man, stood hunched beside Brock's small widow. They, together with several FBI agents, stood watch in the cool morning air as cemetery workers rolled back the artificial grass that covered the new grave. A yellow earth-moving machine began the excavation, scooping up the earth so recently piled on the cement burial vault below. At a distance a gray limousine stood waiting to receive the coffin and transport it to a funeral home in Kalamazoo where the salvaging of tissue would take place.

A pathologist from the VA was to undertake this operation. When the coffin arrived, the lid was opened, the body was lifted onto a table, and the pathologist began the procedure. In the presence of witnesses from the FBI, he made incisions in the body and began to take thin slices from the liver, bladder wall, lungs, and kidneys, placing each specimen into a plastic bag. The bags were then sealed, signed by the pathologist and witnesses, dated, and given into the keeping of the agents. Stored under refrigeration, the bags would be sent to an FBI laboratory in Washington where a forensic chemist would begin to devise the test needed to identify the presence of Pavulon in the tissues.

There were four exhumations during the first week of October. All the deceased were patients whose deaths were judged highly suspicious. In each case the FBI had applied to the families of the patients for permission to disinter the bodies. In the presence of notaries the next of kin had signed affidavits allowing the exhumations to take place. County Health Departments in each of the counties where exhumations were planned issued permits for disinterment and reburial.

With these legal permissions in place, the prosecutor had proceeded to order the exhumations. Now he, and everyone involved, would have to wait for word from the laboratory in Washington.

* * *

In early October the agents began to pack up their files, preparing to move out of the hospital and turn over the results of their investigation to the U.S. Attorney's Office in Detroit.

Jay Bailey, the agent in charge of the FBI office in Detroit, told the *Ann Arbor News*, "This does not mean we are curtailing our efforts or reducing manpower in this investigation." The headquarters in the hospital, he said, had been a convenient place to conduct the bulk of the interviews. "We've now completed all the necessary interviews. We will continue the investigation from our headquarters in Detroit and in our Ann Arbor office."

The departure of the agents was very likely a relief to many hospital employees and especially to the ICU nurses who had felt so beleaguered by the FBI presence. But it was relief tempered by the knowledge that as yet no arrest had been made. It seemed that no suspect had been positively identified. That both Filipina Narciso and Leonora Perez had been reassigned to positions not involving patient care had been noted, of course, but the idea that these reassignments indicated suspicion of guilt seemed preposterous to the nurses' coworkers. That these two women could be involved in anything so ghastly was inconceivable.

PART 2

THE TRIAL

CHAPTER 19

Attorney Thomas O'Brien remembers being called at home the first Sunday morning in October. It was a young associate from his law firm on the line. The firm had received a call from a nurse at the VA, the associate said. She and another nurse were being investigated by the FBI, and apparently the agents were giving them a terrible time. Would O'Brien speak with the nurses?

O'Brien was, of course, aware of the problems at the VA. He had first learned of the situation months earlier when *CBS News* interrupted a scheduled broadcast to announce that the FBI was investigating a series of breathing failures at the hospital. Subsequently news about the situation had become almost inescapable.

In an article written in the 1980s for the journal *Litigation,* O'Brien recounted the events following the call from his associate: "A half hour later, dressed in jeans, I watched two pleasant-looking young Filipino nurses walk down the hall to my office, followed by relatives and small children. It was hard to believe the FBI considered them suspects in some bizarre plot to murder hospital patients."

O'Brien asked the nurses to come into his office. "It turned out that they had been undergoing lengthy interrogations by the FBI for weeks without any sort of legal counsel," he wrote. "They were not yet citizens of the United States and, as federal employees, they felt obligated to cooperate with every demand the FBI made." Narciso told him of her six-hour interrogation and the agents' pressure on her to confess. "That night her roommates and their landlord found her sobbing in her room," O'Brien wrote. "They insisted that she talk to a lawyer."

Narciso had had similar advice from others, advice that she had resisted, saying that in the Philippines an innocent person did not hire a lawyer, but eventually she had been persuaded. "I was the second lawyer she saw," O'Brien wrote. "The first one practiced in Ypsilanti, where she lived. He listened to her impassively for fifteen minutes, gave her a business card and said, 'Call me if they arrest you.'"

O'Brien remembered spending a long time with the nurses that Sunday. In the end he agreed to represent them both. "While it was already an important case," he wrote, "I had no idea what was coming."

O'Brien was a young man that summer. In newspaper photographs taken at the time he appears to be in his early thirties, fit, confident, and remarkably good-looking. A thick shock of hair falling across his forehead gave him an almost boyish air. His article in *Litigation* begins with the sentence, "I always wondered what it would be like to try a big case." On that Sunday in October he could not have foreseen how big a case the *United States of America v. Filipina Narciso and Leonora Perez* was about to become, but he was not long discovering.

On the eighteenth of November the *Detroit Free Press* reported, "The U.S. Attorney's office has opened a federal grand jury investigation into the string of apparent murders and murder attempts that struck the Veterans Administration Hospital in Ann Arbor last summer."

Leonora Perez and Filipina Narciso were the first witnesses subpoenaed to appear before the jury. Neither nurse had been "singled out" as a suspect in the case, O'Brien told the press. A subpoena was merely a summons to appear as a witness. Perez and Narciso were the first to be summoned, O'Brien said, but he understood there would be a number of others.

The object of a grand jury investigation is to determine whether sufficient evidence exists to warrant bringing a case to trial. The proceedings of the investigation take place in a strictly controlled situation. Information obtained from witness testimony is not disclosed unless there is a trial. Jury members are forbidden by law to discuss or report on any part of what they hear in the grand jury chamber. Witnesses appear alone before the jury without the presence of legal counsel.

On a wintry Thursday in November, the two women, accompanied by O'Brien, traveled from Ann Arbor to the federal courthouse in Detroit to comply with the summons. Snow was spitting when they reached the city. The massive government building seemed to loom above the crowded street.

They were shown into a small room where they were to remain until called to appear before the jury. Sitting on straight-backed chairs, they waited. O'Brien would be required to remain in the anteroom while the women testified. If either needed his counsel, she could leave the hearing to speak to him, but he would not be permitted to be present in the grand jury chamber.

Perez was the first to be called. She was questioned for almost three hours. What was asked in those three hours is protected by the secrecy surrounding all grand jury proceedings, but one can assume that the testimony she previously gave to the FBI formed the basis for the questions.

Narciso's appearance began late on Thursday afternoon and was relatively brief. O'Brien told the *Ann Arbor News*, "When Miss Narciso was summoned it was almost the end of the working day so she was asked, and we agreed, to appear in a couple of weeks." Prosecutor Delonis confirmed this, saying, "We didn't have enough time to do everything we wanted to do, so Miss Narciso will be coming back."

It was approaching five o'clock as this day of hearings came to an end. Twilight was already darkening the streets outside the courthouse when the nurses emerged. O'Brien wrote in his *Litigation* account, "[W]e knew that every move they made would be scrutinized by network cameras and seasoned reporters. The familiar image of a grand jury witness covering his head, running from reporters—was a scene we intended to avoid. These women said they were innocent and they looked innocent. That was exactly how they would present themselves. That approach worked. The news accounts described them as pleasant, open, and polite. . . . . Based upon what the government lawyers had told them, (the nurses) did not believe that they had been singled out by the FBI or the grand jury. But they were wrong."

CHAPTER 20

From the beginning of the investigation the FBI agents had been frustrated in their efforts to find eyewitnesses to the events now being presented to the grand jury. The hundreds of interviews they conducted had produced no such witness, and the few leads they followed had resulted in dead ends. If the grand jury decided that a trial was warranted, eyewitness testimony would be vital to the prosecution's case. Yet, improbable as it seemed in a facility the size of the VA, the months of investigation had turned up no one. Only Jordan Olson had provided testimony that seemed promising, but now, of course, Olson was no longer telling the same story.

A psychiatrist the agents consulted about the problem suggested that nurses who might have witnessed suspicious acts were repressing the memory, unwilling to believe that one of their colleagues could be responsible for cold-blooded murder. Another source suggested the possibility of a "curtain of silence"—nurses refusing to testify against one of their own.

Early in December, while the grand jury hearings continued, agents Daniel Russo and Richard Gutler journeyed to western Michigan to meet with Olson in his home, doubtless hoping that time and healing might have restored his original memories of events. With them they brought six photographs of ICU nurses, including pictures of Narciso and Perez. They planned to ask Olson to try to identify the nurse who had given him the paralyzing injection.

When Russo and Gutler reached Olson's home, they found a man pale and clearly weakened but pleasant and willing to cooperate. He studied the photographs the agents showed him and, after a short time, positively identified Perez. She was the nurse who had injected him, he said. He thought he had always insisted that Perez was the one responsible for his arrest. He had no memory of seeing Narciso at his bedside or of giving a note to Dr. Goodenday. He realized, he said, that what he recalled now was different from what he had reported earlier. He couldn't explain the disparity.

The agents asked Olson if he would be willing to undergo hypnosis in an effort to clarify his memories. Hypnosis was a procedure that Delonis and the FBI had only recently begun to consider as a tool for use in the investigation. There was reason to believe that if a session of hypnosis could reactivate patients' memories of events, useful information might be obtained in subsequent interviews. Delonis did not intend to offer transcripts of the sessions themselves as evidence in court. Such material would likely be inadmissible. But testimony taken later from patients whose memories had been reactivated in this way could serve the prosecutor's case. These patients could appear in court to testify.

Hypnosis was an unusual procedure to consider, but there were legal precedents. Delonis had learned of other cases in which hypnosis was used to refresh the memory of a witness and, eager as the US attorneys were to strengthen their case, hypnosis seemed desirable, a possible way to obtain the much-needed eyewitness.

The sessions would be administered under the direction of a qualified medical expert in the field of hypnosis, the agents told Olson. In fact such an expert had already been contacted. Dr. Herbert Spiegel, an associate clinical professor of psychiatry in the College of Physicians and Surgeons at Columbia University in New York City, was a doctor whose impeccable credentials and experience in other court cases involving hypnosis made him ideal for the undertaking. He had agreed to come to Ann Arbor to administer the sessions.

Olson said he was willing to undergo hypnosis if that could help clarify his memory. He signed the form the agents had brought with them, consenting to the procedure.

In mid-December the sessions began. Six former patients who had previously undergone arrests were contacted. Like Olson, they were asked to sign consent forms and return to the hospital to take part in the procedures.

Delonis hoped to attract no attention to the undertaking. The patients were brought to the hospital secretly on the weekend preceding the scheduled sessions. They were sequestered in the north wing on the fifth floor under tight security, and, at the request of the FBI, their names were not recorded in the official list of admissions.

On the sixteenth of December, Dr. Spiegel and three FBI agents met in the room where the sessions were to take place. The agents would assist Spiegel in questioning the patients after Spiegel had succeeded in hypnotizing them. The sessions were to be videotaped.

One of the first patients to be hypnotized was Stuart Neff who had undergone an arrest on the thirtieth of July while watching a televised baseball game. Since his arrest Neff had claimed to have no memory of the events preceding it. He could recall no one in his hospital room at the time. Now, under hypnosis, he was asked to return to that room on that evening in July and to describe what he saw as though he were watching events on a television screen.

Carefully the agents began their questioning, taking pains to word their questions in such a way that they would not seem to be leading Neff or influencing his answers. A transcript of this interview begins with Gutler asking Neff to look at the screen and picture himself in his hospital room. "Are you lying in bed?," Dr. Spiegel asked.

"Uh-huh."

"Can you tell us—what you are seeing and feeling?"

"I feel like shaking the hell out of the side of the bed, hollering for the nurses to come out and see what was the matter with me."

As Spiegel and the agents continued to ask questions, Neff's memory seemed to become increasingly vivid. "They did something to knock me out one night," he said.

An agent asked him to look at the screen and picture somebody who would do something like that. Neff had already mentioned several persons who had been in his room at one time or another before his arrest. Now he said he kind of hated to say it. He didn't want to get anyone in trouble. But on his screen he saw "that one Filipino girl."

Slowly in the answers that followed Neff gave a description of "the Filipino girl" that fit Perez far better than Narciso. She was small, he said, thin, nicely stacked. She had dark hair down to her shoulders, a nice ass. But this nurse didn't like him, Neff said. She wasn't friendly. He remembered calling to her for help, but she didn't help him. She only turned and quickly hurried from his room.

In recalling the episode, Neff seemed almost to be reliving it. When the session ended, he continued to turn his head from side to side as if still looking for the nurse who had been in his room.

When Russo and Gutler interviewed Neff again some weeks later and showed him nurses' photographs, he identified Perez. She was identical to the nurse he had seen exiting his room at the time of his arrest, he said.

It seemed that hypnosis, at least in Neff's case, had accomplished what Delonis and the agents hoped it would. They had an eyewitness.

CHAPTER 21

Early in December Filipina Narciso was summoned to reappear before the grand jury in order to complete her testimony.

For some time O'Brien had been attempting to arrange for her return to active nursing duties. He did not expect either Perez or Narciso to be indicted, he said, and saw no reason that Narciso could not return to her former duties. For Leonora Perez, reinstatement at the Ann Arbor VA was no longer an issue. In the early days of the investigation she had applied for a transfer to a VA hospital in Chicago. Her husband had found work in the area. The couple had relatives and friends there. In November she had obtained the transfer, and shortly thereafter she and her family moved to Illinois.

The US attorneys tried to block the transfer when they learned of it, but O'Brien had managed to intercede, giving assurances that Mrs. Perez would return to Michigan to testify again before the grand jury should she be called.

At both VA hospitals the official word was that the women would not be returned to active nursing duties until their role in the murder investigation was clarified. Immigration officials had taken the same position. The nurses' applications for US citizenship would be put on hold until the outcome of the murder probe was known. No one was predicting when that would be.

In the middle of January, Perez was summoned to reappear before the grand jury. A day or two prior to her return, the *Ann Arbor News* published a front-page story claiming that the US Attorney's Office in Detroit was preparing to ask for criminal indictments against both Narciso and Perez within two weeks. The following day a Detroit paper quoted officials close to the investigation flatly denying the report. Delonis had called it "purely speculative." But on the same day the *News* quoted a second source, confirming the original story: "I'd say your story is quite accurate although your date might be a little premature. Indictments will probably be closer to February 15."

On the fifteenth of January Perez and four or five other VA nurses appeared before the grand jury. If Perez had heard any rumors about pending indictments she gave no indication of it. She was smiling as she emerged from the grand jury room, saying that she had been "asked about some tapes."

Presumably these were tapes made during the hypnosis sessions in December. Among them would likely have been the tape of Neff's session in which he described "that one Filipino girl" in terms that seemed to fit Perez, but Perez said nothing more about what she had been asked.

* * *

The day following Perez's appearance the grand jury adjourned. This did not mean that the jury had finished its investigation, Delonis told the press, saying that the jury would reconvene in a few weeks. The investigation would continue. He had nothing to say about indictments.

While the jury was in recess the papers had little fresh news to report. Other stories began to occupy front pages. But in February the VA investigation was front page news again.

On February 4 Perez and Narciso and sixteen other nurses were served subpoenas ordering them to appear in a lineup at the Police Department in Westland, a town some twenty miles from Ann Arbor. The nurses were to appear dressed in their uniforms. They would be photographed and perhaps fingerprinted at this time.

O'Brien strongly objected, saying that the subpoenas were unreasonable and his clients had been charged with nothing. But his objections did not cancel the order. It seemed that Perez and Narciso would have to appear. On the twelfth of February they set out for Westland.

Waiting in the Westland Police Department were persons who had been called to view the lineup. Among them were several patients who had suffered suspicious arrests during July and August and some of their family members. There were also a few members of the VA staff, several FBI agents, and representatives from the US Attorney's Office.

Of the nurses subpoenaed, as many as fifteen were of Asian origin. Most were currently employed at the VA or recently had been. In Westland they were divided into groups of six.

The nurses, one group at a time, entered the room where they were to stand and faced a wall fitted with a panel of one-way glass. In a room on the other side of the wall the observers took turns viewing the groups while they themselves were concealed behind the glass panel. The FBI had asked the observers to withhold any identification they could make until they had viewed all three groups, saying that the agents would take statements later.

The lineups began at 8:00 p.m. and lasted until almost midnight. Whatever information the FBI gained as a result of this effort was, of course, not made public. An attorney in the prosecutor's office told the *Ann Arbor News* that while the grand jury investigation continued he was prohibited from commenting on any phase of the probe.

CHAPTER 22

Stuart Neff was been among the former patients at the Westland lineup. He was in no condition to make the trip from his home in Indiana his doctors told Delonis. His health had seriously deteriorated in the months since his hypnosis. The doctors did not expect him to live long.

This was a serious blow to the prosecution's case. Should Neff die, the attorneys would lose their chief witness. In fact, his identification of Leonora Perez, made at the FBI interview subsequent to his hypnosis, was the only really reliable, eyewitness testimony the prosecution had.

Although Jordan Olson had also identified Perez in his December interview with the FBI, his testimony was not considered reliable. Thus, Neff's testimony was vital to the prosecution. If he could not appear in court to testify, its case would be seriously weakened. The transcript of the FBI interview would not suffice as evidence if Neff were not present to attest to the truth of what he had told the agents.

With this in mind the government attorneys filed a motion on March 1, asking Judge Philip Pratt of the Federal District Court for permission to take a sworn deposition from Neff. They provided the judge with a physician's affidavit testifying to the severity of Neff's condition. They argued the need to have Neff's sworn testimony available on the court record should the case eventually come to trial. Significantly, and for the first time, Leonora Perez and Filipina Narciso were named as suspects in the case.

O'Brien strenuously objected to the motion. As he wrote later, "We opposed the motion on Constitutional grounds. The Fifth Amendment prohibits the government from holding anyone to answer for a capital crime on anything less than a grand jury finding of cause. In the Constitutional sense, this deposition would force them [the nurses] to defend themselves in a judicial proceeding on mere suspicion." He continued, "Before anyone was indicted, they [the prosecutors] asked for a court order compelling the attendance of the nurses at the deposition. They were described in the motion simply as "suspects of the grand jury."

Delonis was acting on a new ruling handed down only months earlier by the US Supreme Court, permitting prosecutors to take depositions to be used as evidence in criminal cases. Whether a deposition taken in a case in which no indictments had yet been handed down would be allowed as evidence was not certain, but, given Neff's condition, Delonis felt he hadn't time to wait for the grand jury to decide on indictments.

Judge Pratt was a solidly built, graying, middle-aged man. He listened impassively to the attorneys' arguments, and on the twenty-sixth of March he ruled in favor of the prosecution's motion. The ruling was unprecedented. It was, apparently, the first time in US history that a witness in a federal criminal case would be allowed to give testimony against suspects not yet indicted or charged. O'Brien immediately filed an appeal to halt the deposition, but the appeal was denied. The deposition was scheduled for April 22.

It would proceed like an official court hearing, with Delonis questioning and O'Brien cross-examining Neff in the presence of Naricso and Perez. A court reporter would make an official transcript. The proceedings would be videotaped and sound recorded as well. The prosecutors hoped that such sworn testimony, taken in the presence of the accused and including a cross-examination by the defense, would be admissible in court.

On April 13 O'Brien counterattacked. He filed a request in federal court, asking for permission to take a sworn deposition from a patient then in the ICU at the Ann Arbor VA. This patient, Ian Collins, had spoken at length with Neff when both were patients in the hospital about the circumstances surrounding Neff's arrest. He reported a story very different from the one Neff had given the FBI. It was a bearded man, Neff had told Collins. A bearded man was the last person he had seen in his room the night he arrested.

This was important testimony, and O'Brien was in a hurry to have it recorded because Collins, too, was a very sick man. He was scheduled to be flown to California to undergo open-heart surgery. Although the doctors gave him a 15 to 20 percent chance of *not* surviving the operation, they agreed that without surgery he had only months to live. The transfer to California would take place in a very few days. For O'Brien speed was essential.

He was aware that amnesia could follow open-heart surgery as it had in the case of Olson. He felt it was crucial to the defense to have Collins's recollections on record for use in refreshing his memory if there were problems after surgery. He asked for an emergency hearing on his motion, but before the request could be acted on, Collins's condition began to deteriorate. His doctors advised against the added strain of a deposition, and Collins refused to be deposed. He was flown to California soon after with no testimony taken and no certainty that it ever would be.

There were rumors in the hospital that Collins had been railroaded. Apparently he had asked later to speak with O'Brien despite his initial refusal, but hospital officials had not made that possible. Some said this was deliberate. Some said the administration was so eager for an indictment that the meeting between O'Brien and Collins had been purposely blocked.

* * *

Of Neff's deposition O'Brien wrote, "[T]he deposition drew international attention. The government's claim that the women were suspects was given prominent coverage in newspapers and television. Their photographs were displayed in news stories that ran around the world." But there would be no members of the media present at the deposition. That had been established.

On April 22 Neff was taken to a sealed courtroom in the South Bend, Indiana, federal courthouse about a half hour from his home. A frail man, he was described as walking haltingly down the marble corridor to the courtroom, once or twice stopping to steady himself against the wall. An armed policeman stood guard outside the door to the courtroom. Thick paper had been taped over the transom above the door to prevent anyone from observing the proceedings within. Given the tight security surrounding the deposition, it is remarkable that within twenty-four hours the newspapers had stories.

Quoting sources, the papers reported that Neff, responding to questions asked by Delonis, identified Perez as the nurse he remembered. He pointed to her in the courtroom, saying that she was the nurse who had left his room as his arrest began. To identify her for the record, he described the clothes she was wearing—a red jacket over a white turtleneck.

O'Brien's cross-examination lasted almost two hours, with Neff admitting that he had lied in previous statements to the FBI and others. He hadn't wanted to get anyone in trouble, he said. But now he was telling the truth because he was disgusted with himself for lying.

The proceedings began at 10:00 a.m. They ended after four that afternoon. Emerging from the building, Perez told reporters that Neff was "confused about everything."

CHAPTER 23

Late in May, nearly a month after Neff's deposition, the US Attorney's Office received word from the federal laboratory in Washington. The testing of the tissues had been completed. As the newspapers were quick to report, traces of pancuronium bromide, or Pavulon, had been found in the tissues of three of the four patients exhumed in October.

Delonis refused to confirm or deny these reports. "3 of 4 is an excellent batting average, isn't it?," he said, "but at this point all, and I mean *all*, that I can say is that the laboratory tests are in." He would not comment on the findings until they had been presented to the grand jury, he said, but it was obvious to reporters that if traces of pancuronium bromide had been found in the tissues of any of the patients for whom the drug had not been ordered, the prosecution had strong evidence of murder.

On the seventh of June the twenty-three-member panel of jurors was reconvened. A source close to the investigation told the *Ann Arbor News* that the panel had been recalled "to fit together the final bits and pieces of evidence before government prosecutors asked the panel to return indictments in the case."

Contacted for comment, Delonis agreed that the jury would be considering "a potpourri of testimony," but when pressed by reporters to discuss indictments, he denied having any immediate plans, adding, "[I]f you are thinking about camping outside the county clerk's office, you could have a fairly long wait."

In fact the wait was not very long. Ten days after the jury reconvened, Thomas O'Brien received a call at his office. It was a Wednesday afternoon. The caller was Kirk Cheyfitz, the *Detroit Free Press* reporter who had covered the VA story from the beginning. The FBI had scheduled a press conference for 4:00 p.m., Cheyfitz told him.

O'Brien had few doubts about the FBI's reason for scheduling the conference at four in the afternoon, just in time to make the evening news broadcasts, but it puzzled him that he had not been contacted directly if indictments were to be announced.

Putting Cheyfitz on hold, he called Filipina Narciso on another line. He reached her at home. When she awakened from a nap, she told him, the FBI was in her house and she was placed under arrest.

O'Brien said he thought he had established a good working relationship with the US attorneys. He had assured them that if his clients were indicted there would be no need to arrest them. They would cooperate voluntarily as they had on other occasions. Yet at that moment Filipina Narciso was under arrest and the arrest of Leonora Perez was soon to follow.

In Chicago that Wednesday afternoon Leonora Perez and a friend were returning from a shopping trip, heading back to the Lakeside VA Hospital where Perez now worked. Suddenly, she later recalled, a car pulled up in the street and stopped beside them. A man got out. Perez recognized him as an FBI agent from Detroit. "Hi Leonie," he said to her. "Come here. You're under arrest."

"I won't come," she told him.

"If you won't come, we'll drag you."

And so she got into the car. What else could she do?

They took her to the federal building in Chicago and asked her to confess. As she remembers it, "They told me, 'You are in trouble. You are in more trouble than P.I. You are married. You have a family. You have a boy. Why don't you just say P.I. did it?'" Perez refused.

Television news broadcasts that evening carried videotape of Perez's arrest as well as portions of the FBI press conference announcing that the federal grand jury in Detroit had that day returned a sixteen-count indictment. The indictment charged Narciso and Perez with five counts of first-degree murder, ten counts of poisoning with intent to injure, and a single count of conspiracy. A conviction on any one of these counts could result in life imprisonment or worse.

Leonora Perez was four months pregnant at the time of her arrest and the mother of a three-year-old son. To many watching as she was handcuffed and taken into custody, it must have been difficult to believe that she could have been involved in such a series of criminal acts, that either woman, in fact, could be guilty of the charges against them. Yet there on the television screen was a representative of the US government announcing the indictments.

O'Brien remembers that for him there was little sleep that night. Calls kept coming from news organizations, from friends and supporters of the nurses, and from the Philippine embassy in Washington. "Sometime after 3:00 a.m. I dozed off," he said. "Then the phone rang again. 'Yes,' I said. 'It is three in the morning.'" The answer crackled over the telephone line from half a world away. "Mr. O'Brien, this is the Voice of the Philippines Radio Network. You are talking live to 15 million Filipinos. How can the American government charge these two innocent women with these crimes?"

It was a question that was soon being asked widely and persistently as sympathy for the nurses began to swell. At the hospital in Ann Arbor news of the indictment was met with a mixture of disbelief and outrage. The two women "cared too much about people to deliberately and wantonly take a life," a nurse and coworker told the *Ann Arbor News*. "They were railroaded," another nurse said.

Narciso was characterized by those who knew her and her work as "one of the best," a nurse loved by her patients. The hospital authorities, on the other hand, were bitterly criticized. A nurse remembered hearing a hospital official predict that the two women would be "nailed," and the authorities had done just that, she said.

The FBI was criticized as well. The agents had "virtually dragged Narciso out of her house" when they arrested her, according to a nurse interviewed by the *News*. The agents were "out to prove to the American public that the FBI was worth its salt" she said.

In the days that followed this became a recurrent theme. Narciso and Perez were widely viewed as victims of the FBI's need to prove itself and of the hospital administration's determination to bring some closure to the scandal tainting the institution.

CHAPTER 24

Narciso spent the night in jail. The following morning she was taken to Detroit for arraignment. She and O'Brien had conferred the night before about how she would plead before the magistrate. "Rest assured it is not going to be 'guilty,'" O'Brien told reporters who were waiting outside the federal courthouse that morning.

As soon as Narciso appeared, cameras began to flash. Handcuffed and flanked by FBI agents, she seemed calm, almost stoic, to those gathered on the sidewalk. Neatly dressed in a white jacket and dark slacks, she glanced neither right nor left as the agents led her into the building.

Presiding at the arraignment was US Magistrate Barbara Hackett. After some preliminaries she asked Narciso how she wanted to plead to the charges against her. In a firm voice Narciso replied, "I am innocent and on my attorney's advice I stand mute." Accordingly Hackett entered a plea of innocent but proceeded to deny Narciso bail.

O'Brien strongly objected, arguing that Ms. Narciso had appeared whenever she had been required to do so during the investigation and grand jury proceedings. She would come to trial when called, he said. There was no need to keep her incarcerated with no hope of release on bond.

Delonis countered, saying that, short of treason, the charges brought against Narciso were the most serious in the criminal code. He asked that she be held without bond.

Hackett did not alter her original decision. Filipina Narciso would remain in jail.

Some two hours later Leonora Perez appeared before a US magistrate in Chicago. It was a brief appearance. The magistrate set a $500,000 bond for her release, which clearly, in Perez's circumstances, was the equivalent of denying bail. Following the arraignment, Perez, in handcuffs and under guard, was flown to Michigan, where she entered the Washtenaw County jail. There she and Narciso were to remain while they awaited trial.

The trial would begin late in August or September, Delonis told reporters, predicting that it would last several months given the complicated and technical nature of the testimony involved. When questioned about a motive for the crimes, he refused to comment.

The question of motive had been central to any discussion of the crimes from the moment that they were recognized as crimes. Although ideas abounded, none seemed entirely satisfactory. Oddly, Stuart Neff's idea of a wide-ranging conspiracy, expressed later to a psychiatrist, seemed to be suggested in the wording of the indictment itself.

The indictment begins, "That beginning on or about the 1st day of July, 1975 and continuing up to and including the 15th day of August, 1975, . . . Filipina Narciso, a/k/a 'P.I.' and Leonora Perez, a/k/a 'Leonie,' defendants herein, did willfully and knowingly combine, conspire, confederate and agree together, with each other and with diverse other persons to the Grand Jury unknown, to commit the following offenses against the United States of America." From there the indictment went on to list the counts of murder and poisoning.

But who were the diverse other persons unknown to the grand jury? Questioned about this, Delonis would say only the obvious, that the wording indicated the possibility of other persons' involvement. The government would not spend time searching for new leads, he said, unless "such information were brought to the attention of the FBI."

How seriously the US attorneys were considering a wider involvement is not clear. Several newspapers reported that sources close to the investigation had suggested that central to the prosecution's argument for motive would be the outrage felt by numerous members of the nursing staff at the oppressive working conditions in the hospital. The papers cited the nurses' earlier petition to the administration, which had produced little change in those working conditions. They suggested that the crisis that had occurred in the summer of 1975 might be explained as a protest, a macabre, dramatic, and desperate ploy to bring an intolerable situation to the attention of the hospital administration. Were Perez and Narciso part of a larger conspiracy at that time? The wording of the indictment left the question open.

On Monday, the twenty-first of June, Leonora Perez was taken from the Washtenaw County jail and driven to the federal courthouse in Detroit for arraignment. Like Narciso, she declared her innocence and stood mute. Like Narciso, she was denied bond.

O'Brien protested the bond action in both cases, saying it was unnecessary and excessive. The prosecutor countered that since the women were not US citizens and had no ties to the community, they might flee the country if released on bond. Because the United States had no extradition agreement with the Philippines, should the women flee to their homeland they would have escaped the jurisdiction of the court.

These arguments were to continue later in the day. A hearing on the issue of bonds had already been scheduled for the afternoon in District Court before Judge Philip Pratt.

That afternoon Judge Pratt's courtroom was packed. More than 150 spectators jammed the room. Still more stood clustered in the hall outside. Most said they were there in support of Narciso and Perez. A large number were Filipino.

O'Brien, in an effort to counter the prosecution's arguments for denying bail, had secured six witnesses who agreed to testify to the women's good character and reliability, aiming to cast doubt on the idea that freed on bond they would flee. Filipina Narciso's Ypsilanti landlord was one of the first of these witnesses to testify. Using Narciso's nickname, he said, "P.I. is a fine girl in every respect." She was "one of the few people in the world" he trusted to care for his young son, his only child. Narciso had once taken the boy alone to northern Michigan to pick cherries. They often went to the movies together. He never worried.

O'Brien asked if he would still trust Narciso with his son. The man replied, "If P.I. were home tonight, I would like very much for him to be able to go to the movies with her."

The theme of trust and admiration continued. An intern who had worked with Perez at the VA claimed that she was an excellent nurse and he had never seen her mistreat a patient. A nursing supervisor, Betty Jakim, said that both women had very fine characters and were "superior to excellent" in their professions. A former patient, asked whether he would trust Narciso to care for him, answered, "Absolutely. I have more confidence in that lady than in my own wife in that kind of situation."

Then he added, "Of course, I wouldn't say that if my wife was here." The spectators burst into laughter.

It appeared that the witnesses had done what O'Brien hoped they would. All six had said they felt the women would not flee the country if freed on bond. They had given glowing reports about the women's characters and their reliability.

But the afternoon was waning, and there had been no decision on the issue. At four-thirty the hearing adjourned. The spectators began dispersing. Handcuffed and shackled together, Narciso and Perez were led away to be returned to the Washtenaw County jail.

CHAPTER 25

The indictment of the nurses was attracting significant attention in the Philippines. O'Brien's 3:00 a.m. phone call was only the beginning. In Manila the indictments made headlines.

Mario Belisario, the chargé d'affaires at the Philippine embassy in Washington, soon reported that his government was protesting the "excessive bail conditions" set for the two women. Very shortly diplomatic notes were delivered to the American embassy in Manila and to the State Department in Washington, requesting that the two nurses be released from jail pending the outcome of the trial. Belisario acknowledged that such diplomatic communication over the handling of a criminal case was unusual, but the case was unusual, he said.

The Philippine foreign secretary had ordered the Philippine consul in Chicago to request that the nurses not be handcuffed as such restraints were not a part of the Philippine process of justice before there was a conviction. Further, he ordered the consul to secure copies of the patient records and charts that were to be used at the trial and have them sent to the Philippine Department of Foreign Affairs in Manila.

Ferdinand Marcos, then president of the Philippines, appointed his brother to head a national campaign to raise money for the nurses' defense. Two well-known Filipino lawyers, one the president of the Philippine Bar Association and one a former senator and Supreme Court justice, had offered their services to the nurses free of charge and were preparing to fly to Detroit. The vice-consul in Chicago announced that either he or the consul general would be present throughout the forthcoming trial as official government observers, intending to demonstrate the Philippine government's support.

In the government-controlled Philippine press, feeling was running high. The nurses were termed scapegoats. Their prosecution was likened to a lynching. Columnists charged racism and claimed that the case was an attempt to discredit foreign workers. Newspapers questioned the competence of the law firm representing the women. They questioned the American system of justice.

This uproar arose at a time when the US and Philippine governments were engaged in sensitive diplomatic negotiations about the future of two major US military bases in the Philippines. Both Clark Air Force Base and Subic Bay Naval Base were located on Luzon, the largest of the Philippine Islands, just off the South China coast. Both were of significant importance to the American presence in the Pacific. Ironically, critical to the negotiations was the question of the Philippine government's jurisdiction over the sixteen thousand Americans and their families stationed at the bases. Although diplomats on both sides denied that the pending prosecution of the nurses would affect the negotiations, it was easy to read the hostility toward the United States expressed in the Philippine press as a reflection of the views of the Marcos government.

Delonis, when questioned by the *Detroit Free Press* about the situation in the Philippines, stolidly refused to change course. Despite the publicity and diplomatic messages, he would not alter his approach or retreat from his position. "Until there's some word from elsewhere [presumably the Department of Justice] it's not going to change me any," he said.

Accordingly, when the hearing resumed on Thursday afternoon, Delonis argued against a release on bond. Because the United States had no extradition agreement with the Philippine government, "It would be quite tempting," he said, "for the defendants to seek refuge, a haven, their freedom that lies but a short distance away by a 747 at Metro airport."

"The government is missing the point," an attorney for the defense replied. "The question should be *will* these two people flee." The defense evidently believed that its character witnesses had established the nurses' reliability in that matter, but there seemed to be no changing the mind of the prosecution.

As the afternoon wore on, the crowd of spectators in the courtroom waited expectantly for a decision from Judge Pratt as to the granting of bail. A decision had been anticipated by the end of that afternoon's hearing, but none was forthcoming. Judge Pratt declared that he would notify the attorneys for the prosecution and the defense when he had made his decision but would not call an open court session to announce it, doubtless disappointing the spectators who had spent two long afternoons hoping for an outcome in the nurses' favor.

At the end of the hearing that day, O'Brien officially withdrew from representation of Perez. This was in conformity with the American Bar Association's rules and ethics. The same attorney could not represent two clients charged with the same crime at trial, and so attorneys Edward Stein of Ann Arbor and Laurence Burgess of Detroit would represent Perez from then on. O'Brien and his partner, Michael Moran, would continue to represent Narciso. The attorneys from the Philippines who had offered their services would act as volunteers, O'Brien said, a "reservoir of expertise." But they would not take part in the trial, lacking the credentials required to serve in a US court of law.

CHAPTER 26

Late the following Monday afternoon Judge Pratt handed down his decision. He set bonds for the nurses at $75,000 apiece, specifying that each woman would be required to put up only 10 percent of her bond, or $7,500, in order to be released.

In addition Pratt set a number of conditions. If the bonds were posted and the women released, they would be required to surrender their passports to a court official and to report to this official every seven days. They would be required to live in Washtenaw or Wayne County and were prohibited from traveling outside them. Some person or organization was to be responsible for regular contact with the defendants and must notify the court immediately if either woman by word or action gave any indication that she might flee.

In explaining his decision, Pratt acknowledged that the danger of flight was real but not so strong a possibility that bail should be denied. He noted that the women had a record of voluntarily appearing in court when required. Although they knew the investigation was focused on them, they had made no attempt to flee.

Mario Belisario, speaking from the Philippine embassy in Washington, called the new bond "really very reasonable," adding that the Philippine government, as a matter of policy, would not contribute money to fund the nurses' defense.

Money was an obvious problem. Besides the $7,500 each woman would need to obtain her release from jail, there would be legal expenses in the upcoming months that could be enormous. As nurses, the women were not highly paid. Their families had limited means. But already there were a number of groups engaged in raising money for the defense.

In Ann Arbor the Narciso-Perez Legal Defense Committee was at work. The Philippine Nurses Association in Manila began collecting funds, as did the Philippine Nurses Association of America in Chicago. A defense committee comprised of nurses at the Ann Arbor VA had been organized months earlier. Now similar groups began to spring up in other parts of the United States, including Atlanta, Nashville, New York, and San Francisco, as well as some cities in Canada. In the Philippines schoolchildren were contributing tiny amounts to a fund to help the nurses.

On the Tuesday following Judge Pratt's decision, the coordinator of the Narciso-Perez Legal Defense Committee reported that her group could post the needed $15,000 that day, saying, "Today is Mrs. Perez' birthday and this would make an excellent gift, I think."

And so on Wednesday, the thirtieth of June, attorneys for the defense presented the court with a certified check for $15,000. Federal marshals removed the women's restraints. But before Judge Pratt granted their release, he asked them to stand before the bench. "You should be aware," he said, "that many people have sacrificed for you, and they must not be disappointed." He asked the women to assure him that they would abide by the conditions of their release.

Outside the federal courthouse reporters and television crews crowded the sidewalks. In the building's lobby friends waited anxiously. "It reminds me of an airport," one woman told the *Ann Arbor News*. "All these people moving around, coming and going. It's just like going to an airport to wait for somebody. Only nobody knows what time the plane is going to land."

Then Narciso and Perez, flanked by their attorneys, walked into the lobby, freed of the handcuffs and restraints that had shackled them together. A wave of cheering and laughter exploded in the room. Friends swarmed around them. Smiling, the women started across the lobby. Neither would discuss the charges against them or what still lay ahead when reporters approached, saying only that they were very happy. They wanted to go home. Then they hurried out of the building and, dodging cameras and reporters, crossed the street to the cars waiting to take them there.

In the weeks that followed the plight of the nurses continued to make news. Few days passed without one or two articles in the local papers reporting on their situation. Late in August the two women agreed to speak publicly about what they had been through. Perez spoke to *Free Press* writer Kirk Cheyfitz about the day of her arrest and the terrible experience this had been for her husband and her son. She could not explain to the boy what had happened, she said. He was too young. But he had not been too young to see his mother arrested and handcuffed on the television screen. "You can't erase it from his mind," she said.

Filipina Narciso spoke with John Barton of the *Ann Arbor News*, describing the six hours of interrogation by the FBI and the pressure to confess exerted by both the agents and the VA chief of staff, Martin Lindenauer: "He told me, 'Why don't you just do what the FBI wants you to do?'" He spoke to her several times about confessing, she said, suggesting that she admit her guilt and say it was a mistake she had made, giving the wrong medication. "I told him I didn't do anything, why should I confess? . . . Then he got mad and I just walked out," she said.

In a subsequent letter to the *Ann Arbor News* Lindenauer denied the allegations, saying that the article was without foundation.

CHAPTER 27

Originally the US attorneys wanted the trial of the nurses to begin in September, but Perez's pregnancy presented a problem. As prosecutor Delonis had predicted, the trial promised to be a long one. Perez was already in her sixth month. If the trial began in September it would in all likelihood be interrupted by the birth of the child and whatever time Perez required to recover from it. Judge Pratt, who would preside at the trial, was concerned about Perez's having to deal with a near-term pregnancy and a trial simultaneously. He was concerned, too, about the jurors and how to keep them innocent of the relentless publicity surrounding the trial during any hiatus. By the first of the year the birth and recovery would have been accomplished and there would be no need for interruption. Pratt set the opening date for January 4.

The delay served the defense attorneys well. Perez's lawyers, Stein and Burgess, had come relatively recently to the case. There was a great deal of material for them to study before the case came to trial. It may be that the delay served the prosecutors, too.

A few days prior to the nurses' release on bond, one of the government's most important witnesses had suffered a fatal heart attack. Jordan Olson was dead. Although Olson's account of the events surrounding his respiratory arrest had changed several times and his original identification of Narciso was no longer so persuasive, it was possible the prosecution could have argued that the changes were the result of amnesia following his heart surgery and did not cancel his original identification. They had the scrawled note he had given to Dr. Goodenday. They had transcripts of FBI interviews conducted at different times that seemed to implicate both nurses. But whether any of this material could be admitted as evidence now that Olson could not testify was in doubt. Certainly the attorneys for the defense would argue that it should not be admitted.

In question, too, were the videotapes of Stuart Neff's deposition. Judge Pratt, in allowing the deposition to be taken before indictments were handed down, had made no ruling as to whether the tapes could be admitted as evidence. Again it was certain that Perez's attorneys would argue against their admission on the grounds that no indictments had been in place at the time the testimony was taken. Thus, Neff's identification of Perez was in jeopardy and the prosecution stood to lose the recorded testimony of its one remaining eyewitness.

Delonis, faced with this situation, requested the court's permission to take a second deposition from Neff. The legal aspects of the case had changed, he argued. Indictments now existed. It was possible that Neff would not live much longer, and surely he was too ill to appear at a trial.

On these grounds Judge Pratt approved a second deposition over the objections of the defense attorneys, who argued that Neff's testimony was and would be tainted. They contended that the FBI agents who had questioned Neff during his hypnosis had introduced suggestions that would influenced any later testimony. The FBI had tampered with his mind. Attorney Stein proposed that in hypnosis "not only can things be brought out of the mind, but things can be put in as well." Arguing that Neff had a history of memory loss and suggestibility, the defense asked the court to order that Neff undergo a complete psychiatric evaluation. Stein said, "The FBI was permitted a look into this man's mind, and, in all fairness, the defense would like a peek, too."

Judge Pratt had seen the tapes of Neff's hypnosis. "It is arguable," he said, "that Mr. Neff may have been rendered more amenable to suggestion by these techniques and that certain lines of questioning may have suggested answers to him while he was in this altered state of consciousness."

Pratt ruled that the defense attorneys' request for a psychiatric evaluation was reasonable and they could choose a psychiatrist for the undertaking, but the deposition would go forward. It was set for October 7, would take place in the South Bend courthouse, and would proceed much as the first one had. Or so the prosecutors expected.

At nine-thirty on the morning of the seventh, attorneys for both the defense and the prosecution were in the courtroom, as were two FBI agents, a court reporter, and the technicians who would tape the proceedings. Neither Perez or Narciso was in the room, nor in South Bend for that matter.

Perez, now in the eighth month of pregnancy, was following the advice of her doctor, who felt a trip to Indiana might cause premature labor and a risky delivery. Narciso, not being directly involved in Neff's testimony and not legally bound to appear, had remained in Michigan as well. "It was as if the prosecution was giving a party and nobody came," an observer remarked.

One of the attorneys for the defense described Delonis as livid. Certainly he was far from happy, frustration plain to see on his usually impassive face. "[E]verything was set and ready to do," he said. "[T]he deposition was supposed to start at 9:30, and at 9:30 and five seconds I learn the defendants are not going to be there." It was almost as if the defense were concealing the fact that the nurses would not appear, he said. But the defense attorneys said simply that they were under no legal obligation to notify the prosecutors that the defendants would be absent.

Lacking defendants, the deposition proceeded. The taping began. But clearly there would be no dramatic moment to match the one recorded on the earlier tape. Neff would not turn to point at Perez.

CHAPTER 28

Any hope that the nurses' trial would actually begin on the fourth of January began to dim in the last weeks of November. Attorneys for the defense had filed a number of pretrial motions. The hearings required to deal with these could not be scheduled in the time remaining before the holidays, and jury selection could not begin until Judge Pratt had ruled on the motions. The trial date was reset for February 1.

On the twenty-eighth of December the pretrial hearings began, beginning with a defense motion to dismiss ten of the sixteen counts listed in the grand jury's indictment. While snow fell on the streets of Detroit, the attorneys in Judge Pratt's courtroom began their arguments.

The nurses had been charged with conspiracy and five counts of murder under federal law. The ten counts of poisoning were based on state law, a Michigan statute making it illegal to "knowingly and unlawfully mingle a poison in intravenously administered food and medicine."

The defense attorneys argued that the federal court had no jurisdiction over state law and that the grand jury had incorrectly invoked the Michigan statute to charge Narciso and Perez with the poisonings. Federal prosecution, they argued, could be based on state law only in cases where acts committed on federal property were not covered by federal law. Federal law existed, they contended, under which the women could be charged.

Richard Yanko, an attorney for the prosecution, disagreed. Federal statutes were more general, he said, and "they just refer to assaults upon a person." Because of the specificity of the Michigan statute, it had been chosen for the charges.

But there was another difference between the statutes, a defense attorney pointed out. The Michigan law called for a maximum penalty of life imprisonment while the federal assault statutes carried sentences of only five years.

A series of complicated arguments ensued. An attorney from the US Department of Justice, called in to aid the prosecution, joined in these, contending first that a federal statute could have been used and then that federal assault law was inappropriate because it did not specifically address the act of poisoning.

Judge Pratt was clearly growing impatient. "You can't have your cake and eat it, too," he said. "You can't say in one breath that you could have charged under the federal assault statute and then come back and say Congress did not include poisoning under that federal statute." He would have to hear any additional legal briefs, he said, before making his decision.

In the meantime there were other hearings scheduled on the admissibility of evidence that the prosecution planned to introduce at the trial.

One was a hearing to consider admitting the tape of Neff's first deposition. A second would be concerned with admission of the note Olson had written naming "PIA."

As expected, the defense objected to admitting Neff's testimony on the grounds that FBI agents had planted ideas in Neff's mind during his hypnosis. To demonstrate the point, the defense asked that the videotape of the session be shown in court. The attorneys had brought in Dr. Martin Orne, a psychiatrist and well-known expert in the field of hypnosis, to testify for the defense.

On the fourth of January, in the darkened courtroom, the tape made during Neff's hypnosis was projected onto a large screen. Neff, sitting in a reclining chair, was encircled by FBI agents. When asked by the agents to describe the events and individuals he could remember in his room just prior to his arrest, Neff mentioned several people: two nursing assistants, a "stocky, black fellow" who kept looking at his "jug of medicine," and "a little Filipino girl." At this juncture Dr. Orne stopped the tape to comment. The agents seemed to be concentrating their attention on the "little Filipino girl," he pointed out, though Neff had mentioned others.

Repeatedly Orne stopped the tape to discuss the cues and suggestions he felt the agents were providing. Neff's story was a "confabulation," he said, made up of suggestions for which a memory was missing. In their stress on certain aspects of Neff's story, the agents could be leading him in a particular direction.

In summing up their arguments that afternoon both for and against the admission of Neff's testimony, the lawyers were eloquent, but Judge Pratt gave no indication as to how he would rule. The next day the hearing moved on to consideration of Olson's note.

The defense was seeking to bar the note from evidence, arguing that it was hearsay. Because Olson could not be present to testify, they argued, admission of the note would violate the confrontation clause in the Sixth Amendment to the Constitution. As O'Brien remembers it, a good deal of time was spent on the legal issue, and then, he said, there was a surprising discovery.

In December Judge Pratt had ordered the prosecution to provide the defense with all the FBI reports covering the statements of potential government witnesses. The defense had subsequently received copies of the reports, but not the original documents. Now, beginning his examination of an FBI witness on that January morning, O'Brien asked for the originals. "He gave them to me," O'Brien later wrote. "I took them to the other members of the defense team so that they could look at them as I questioned the witness. In a few moments I could tell that something was causing a lot of discussion at the defense table."

The attorneys at the defense table had discovered that information contained in the original documents had been deleted from the copies in their possession. Missing from the copied reports were statements made by Olson on three occasions claiming that the woman he identified as PIA was an American nurse, a Caucasian. Missing as well was a claim that he did not recall giving a note to Dr. Goodenday nor agreeing to undergo hypnosis in an attempt to straighten out his various versions of events. From the copy of an interview the agents had conducted with an intern, Olson's naming of a male nurse as his attacker had been deleted. Paragraphs had been rearranged in the copies in an apparent attempt to conceal the redactions.

The defense attorneys were outraged. Clearly what had been deleted from the copies of the original documents was material helpful to the defense of the nurses, a violation of established legal principles.

Basic to American law is the principle that attorneys for both the prosecution and the defense are bound to serve the cause of justice. In adherence to this principle, prosecutors are obliged to disclose to the defense any evidence that might establish the innocence of the accused. It was clear that the government attorneys had attempted to circumvent this obligation.

"We asked for a recess," O'Brien wrote, "and informed the court of this development." Retiring to Judge Pratt's chambers, they accused Delonis of deliberately and improperly withholding information and thus denying the nurses a fair trial.

Delonis admitted that the FBI reports had been redacted and some material excised, but he insisted this was not improper. At the time the reports were turned over to the defense, he said, the court had not yet ruled on whether the defense attorneys should have free access to the interviews.

Judge Pratt appeared unmoved by the explanation. He had ordered all material turned over. Now, in no uncertain terms, he again ordered Delonis to turn over to the defense complete transcripts of all the interviews the FBI had conducted together with any other relevant material that had been withheld. When O'Brien and Stein left the courthouse late that afternoon, they were carrying an armload of newly acquired documents. The next morning, citing prosecutorial misconduct, they asked the court to dismiss the case.

Judge Pratt did not rule for a dismissal, although he acknowledged that he could see merit in the request given the prosecution's actions. Instead, after several hours spent consulting with the attorneys in his chambers, he returned to the courtroom, looking weary, and announced an indefinite postponement of all court proceedings in the case in order to give the defense attorneys sufficient time to study the material that had been withheld from them.

O'Brien wrote, "After a lengthy FBI and grand jury investigation, with virtually no information passing to the defense, we finally had the chance to take the offensive. While the factual discovery that came from the hearings assisted in our defense preparations, putting the government on the defensive also gave us some momentum as the trial approached."

CHAPTER 29

Clearly Judge Pratt was greatly influenced by the prosecutors' actions in redacting the FBI reports. The following day he issued an order strictly limiting the evidence the government attorneys could present at trial. This was in response to the attorneys' request to introduce into evidence twenty-four additional breathing arrests involving patients whose names did not appear in the indictment. Doing this would significantly expand the number of criminal attacks that could be included in the conspiracy charge. Pratt's order effectively blocked the strategy, but, as soon became apparent, the prosecution found a way around the order. On the first of February, when the hearings resumed, the defense attorneys discovered that they were faced with a new indictment.

The previous day the federal grand jury had been reconvened to consider new charges brought by the prosecution. Late that afternoon the jury issued an indictment that canceled the first, replacing the charge of conspiracy to commit murder with a charge stating that the nurses had conspired to injure patients at the VA by poisoning. Three of the five murder counts listed as overt acts in the original indictment had been dropped, as had two of the original ten counts of poisoning, but fourteen additional patients who had undergone arrests were named as victims in the conspiracy count.

US Attorney Philip Van Dam, who had replaced Delonis as head of the prosecution team, did not explain the request for a new indictment, but the reason seemed obvious to the defense. O'Brien called it an effort by the government attorneys to make "an end run" around Judge Pratt's order. It appeared, he said, that the prosecutors had taken the names of patients the judge had told them they could not include because they did not appear in the original indictment and simply added them to the new one.

This maneuver can only have further stoked the defense attorneys' outrage at the prosecution's tactics. Of the fourteen new patients listed in the indictment, they objected to three in particular and asked Judge Pratt to strike them.

The hearings continued for another ten days, taking up the motions to bar Stuart Neff's testimony and Olson's note from evidence. By the time the attorneys began their final arguments, the pretrial hearings had consumed the better part of two months.

In his final argument O'Brien accused the prosecution of "foot dragging" and intending to disobey the orders of the court. The defense stated that if the three disputed charges contained in the new indictment were allowed to stand, the attorneys for the defense would be forced to ask for an adjournment while they investigated the charges, further delaying the beginning of the trial.

Van Dam countered that the defense had been offered the names and medical files of all fifty-one patients who had undergone breathing arrests in the hospital but had chosen to look at only those mentioned in connection with their clients. He said that he did not think the court had the authority to strike charges from the indictment.

But on the twelfth of February Pratt did just that, striking all three charges. He ruled that Olson's note could not be admitted as evidence because there was no possibility of cross-examination. But he did not exclude Stuart Neff's testimony from evidence. The trial jury could determine Neff's credibility, he said.

The defense had won several rounds that day, but its failure to win a dismissal of Neff's testimony still presented serious problems. There was no knowing how a jury would judge his credibility or how it would assess FBI influence on what he had to say. His identification of Perez remained of grave concern to her attorneys.

And then, suddenly, Neff's testimony was no longer a problem. Although the government attorneys had argued strenuously for permission to obtain his depositions and admit his testimony into evidence, and Neff was the only living witness to have identified either nurse, the prosecution abruptly and with little explanation dropped his name from the indictment.

Van Dam would say only that this action was in the best interest of the case. Evidently the government attorneys felt that Neff's testimony, filled as it was with confusion and inconsistencies, would, if presented to the jury, do little to advance their case and could, in fact, weaken it overall. Others have suggested that the government dropped Neff from the indictment in order to protect the FBI from charges of improper questioning techniques. Certainly the defense intended to make this charge at the trial and might thus have cast doubt on the credibility of other testimony contained in the FBI reports.

Whatever the prosecution's reason, removing Neff's name from the indictment reduced to eleven the number of overt acts charged against the nurses. Yet the fact remained that conviction on any one of these would likely result in life imprisonment.

CHAPTER 30

Now that Judge Pratt's rulings were in place and the hearings were at an end, the trial of the nurses could go forward. Jury selection was scheduled to begin on the first of March.

No one thought that selecting a jury for this trial would be swift or easy. The extensive media coverage surrounding the VA poisonings from the outset was bound to complicate the process. It was assumed that most of the prospective jurors would have knowledge of the case against the nurses and many would have formed opinions. It was up to the judge and the attorneys to select a jury of fair-minded men and women who could render a verdict based on the evidence presented, a verdict untainted by bias or preconceptions.

Predicted to last two weeks, the selection continued for nearly four. Judge Pratt and the attorneys screened well over one hundred prospective jurors before they arrived at the sixteen they needed—twelve to be impaneled and four to serve as alternates should illness or other contingency require a juror to leave the panel.

On the morning selection began the potential jurors were assembled in a room in the federal courthouse in Detroit. They were men and women of many ages and backgrounds whose names had been culled at random from voter registration rolls in the state. Summoned for duty, they were required by law to appear.

They had filled out forms answering questions about themselves and their occupations, which would be made available to the attorneys. They had received information about the jury process. Now they sat, waiting. Some fidgeted impatiently. Others leafed through the limp pages of old magazines they found in the room. A few dozed, stretched out in their chairs and cushioning their heads on their clasped hands. They had been told that they would be divided into groups of twenty and eventually led, group by group, into the courtroom for questioning, but so far nothing seemed to be happening. Fidgeting or dozing, they waited.

When the clerk of the court finally appeared in the doorway, there was a stir of anticipation. The clerk was holding a plain wooden box. From the box, he told them, he would draw names, aiming to divide the crowd into groups of twenty. Reaching into the box, he pulled out a slip of paper, glanced at it, and called out the first name.

Meanwhile, in the courtroom, the judge, the attorneys, the defendants, and some fifty spectators were assembling to await the first group of twenty. Judge Pratt took his place at the bench. Seated at separate tables facing the bench were the several attorneys for the defense and prosecution, as well as Perez and Narciso. Behind the tables, in a section reserved for spectators, members of the nurses' families were finding seats. They had been flown to Detroit at the expense of a Philippine airline. Quietly they settled themselves.

When the first group of twenty prospective jurors entered, the courtroom quieted. Led to the jury box, this group was seated only long enough to hear the judge enumerate the charges against Perez and Narciso. Then they were led away again to wait in a nearby room. They would be called individually for questioning.

And so the process began. The first prospective juror was brought back into the courtroom and seated. Judge Pratt began his questions. "Had this man read or heard about the case?," he asked. "Had he formed opinions about it? Had he served in the military? Was he familiar with VA hospitals? What was his attitude toward persons of other nationalities?"

In this initial questioning any individual who expressed obvious bias or seemed unlikely to maintain objectivity was excused from serving. Those who had made it through Judge Pratt's forty or fifty questions and were retained were then given over to the attorneys for more questioning.

The selection of jurors was of extreme importance to the attorneys. A case could be won or lost depending on how carefully a jury was chosen. Often lawyers will hire a jury consultant to advise them on the suitability of one or another individual.

Each attorney could challenge a prospective juror for cause, asking for his or her dismissal on the basis of answers that the attorney felt indicated some factor inimical to his case. But dismissal for cause depended on Judge Pratt's agreeing to the challenge. Each attorney had, in addition, twenty-two peremptory challenges for which there was no requirement to show cause.

These challenges were based on the attorney's assessment of the prospective juror, an almost psychological appraisal of how well or badly the individual would serve his case. Would the housewife from the suburbs be likely to feel sympathy for Leonora Perez and her newborn son? Was the old man from Dearborn too timid to maintain his position if it conflicted with the positions of others on the panel? A peremptory challenge is partly a guess, partly a decision made intuitively or with the aid of a consultant.

By the eighth day seventy prospective jurors had been reviewed, but only fourteen had been selected to serve. Often when the number neared sixteen, a peremptory challenge reduced the count and, as the newspapers reported, the endeavor dragged on.

And then, on the thirteenth of March, as the selection was about to enter its third week, the *Detroit Free Press* reported shocking news. "Nurse, Now Dead, Claimed She Poisoned VA Patients" read the headline on the front page of the Sunday edition. On an inner page there was another headline: "Nurse Confessed to VA Slayings, Later Killed Herself."

The case had often been called bizarre. Suddenly the word seemed hardly sufficient.

CHAPTER 31

Betty Jakim was a small, soft-spoken woman who had worked as a nurse for a number of years at the Ann Arbor VA. During the summer of 1975 she had been the nursing supervisor on the three-thirty to midnight shift.

Like almost everyone working in the hospital that summer, Jakim had been interviewed by the FBI. For a time she was considered a possible suspect because of her presence in the hospital during the hours in which the arrests were occurring. As a supervisor, she had unquestioned access to all parts of the building and was one of only two workers on the night shift who had access to the hospital pharmacy after hours. It seemed that she had both the means and the opportunity to commit the crimes, but she was eventually dropped from the list of possible suspects. She had not been in the hospital *every* time a breathing arrest occurred, as Perez and Narciso had been.

At that time Jakim was being treated for cancer, receiving periodic injections of a drug that caused great variations in her mood. Shortly after an injection she appeared almost euphoric to her coworkers, but as the effects of the drug lessened she became listless and depressed and at these times seemed unsympathetic to patients. The ICU was her "vegetable patch" she had told an FBI agent during her interview. The patients were her "little vegetables," and she had more than once remarked that she saw no point in the lifesaving emergency measures so often employed that summer.

Twice during these periods of depression Jakim had attempted suicide. In the summer of 1976, after one of these attempts, she was admitted to the University of Michigan's Neuropsychiatric Institute, where she was diagnosed as suffering from severe depression, acute guilt feelings, and periodic hallucinations. Although only recently she had testified as a character witness at Perez and Narciso's bond hearing, now she was being judged seriously mentally ill.

It was while she was a patient at the institute that she began to claim repeatedly that she was responsible for the deaths at the VA. A number of nurses and other medical personnel had heard her make these statements but had evidently dismissed them as delusions. In any case no information about these statements seems to have been reported to anyone in authority.

Jakim was treated with medication and electric shock therapy. After some months of treatment her symptoms began to grow milder, although she continued to suffer feelings of guilt. At the end of the year she was released from the institute. Soon after she and her husband left for Florida, where they owned a home, and it was there, on the third of February, that Betty Jakim died, having overdosed on tranquilizers prescribed for depression.

When word of her suicide reached Ann Arbor, many of the nurses and other personnel at the Neuropsychiatric Institute recalled her statements while a patient there. A month or so after her death a psychiatric worker (who was later suspended from his job for breach of confidence) spoke with a reporter from the *Detroit Free Press*, recounting Jakim's frequent claims of responsibility for the VA murders. He reported her saying, "Oh my God, I really did it!" Her claims were common knowledge in the hospital, he said.

When the *Free Press* article appeared, the reaction was intense and immediate. The defense attorneys declared that if the prosecution had withheld evidence concerning Jakim they would file again to dismiss the case, and it seemed possible that Judge Pratt would look favorably on such a motion given the prosecution's earlier failure to comply with his orders for disclosure. The government attorneys vowed that they had known nothing about Jakim's claims until they read about them in the *Free Press*, but the defense was not mollified. The defense attorneys issued a subpoena for all Jakim's medical records and demanded any FBI material concerning her that they had not received. Judge Pratt arranged a conference to attempt to determine whether or not evidence had been withheld. It was too soon to know how these new developments would affect the case against the nurses, but nonetheless jury selection continued, moving into its third week.

The day after the *Free Press* story appeared, Prosecutor Van Dam dispatched FBI agents to Florida. Evidently Jakim had written a note before she died, which remained in her husband's possession. He was refusing to show it to the police or other authorities. The few friends who had seen it declared that it contained no admission of guilt, only an insistence on the nurses' innocence, but Van Dam wanted it.

In the middle of the week that followed the defense learned that the university was refusing to comply with the subpoena for Jakim's medical records. Appearing in court, attorneys for the University of Michigan and its Neuropsychiatric Institute argued that the records contained communications between a psychiatrist and a patient and that the confidential nature of those communications was protected by law. Violating this confidentiality, they argued, would destroy the trust necessary in treating mental patients.

This argument did not satisfy the press or many others in the surrounding communities. A *Free Press* editorial published on the twenty-second of March declared that the instinctive reaction to the university's refusal to release the records was "a sense of outrage." The writer conceded that, given the law, the university was doing the only thing it could but argued that the fate of the nurses might hinge on information contained in the hospital records. The law should be changed, the editorial continued, so as to allow this right of privileged communication to be revoked by court order.

Many people agreed. The university's refusal to release the records was hard to accept. If Mrs. Jakim's medical records could exonerate the nurses, some way should be found to circumvent the law.

The psychiatric worker who had spoken to the *Free Press* reporter summed up his feelings quite simply: "Mrs. Jakim is dead—two other lives are involved—you have to make a moral judgement."

Mrs. Jakim's husband had given the federal authorities permission to introduce his wife's records in court. Whether or not this permission had weight with the university's lawyers is unclear. Nor is it clear why the records were finally released to Judge Pratt, although it seems this must have been in response to a court order. In any case, as O'Brien wrote, the judge eventually permitted the attorneys to review the records, first ruling that what they found there was subject to a protective order and could not be used as evidence. O'Brien says that the contents were never disclosed.

But the content of one of Mrs. Jakim's notes *was* made public by the U.S. attorneys. She had written at least two that her husband turned over to the government. The one made public had been written just prior to her hospitalization. In it she declared, "Never did I harm a patient, nor do I believe Pia and Leonie did," which obviously cast doubt on her later claims.

But in fact there was little to validate these claims, or at least little that could be used in court. The claims were only hearsay, statements made by a mentally ill woman who could not, herself, testify to their validity. Thus, in less than ten days what had seemed a possibly important development in the case had become little more than a curious footnote.

CHAPTER 32

After an investigation that had lasted ten months and was rumored to have cost the US government close to a million dollars, after further months of pretrial hearings and weeks of jury selection whose scope had set an unofficial record in the Detroit Federal District Court, and after a full nineteen months had passed since the poisonings in the VA were initially suspected, the trial of the nurses was finally scheduled to begin.

The government opened its case on a rainy morning at the end of March. Shortly before nine o'clock the two teams of attorneys and the defendants entered the courtroom and settled at their respective tables. The room was beige walled and windowless. Nothing in it suggested that taxpayers' dollars had been spent on appearance or comfort. The spectators, already gathered, sat on plain wooden benches at the back of the room. The attorneys' tables were stolid, dark wood structures illuminated by glaring overhead lights.

Next the jurors filed in, ten women and six men. There was an audible stir among the spectators as they took their places in the jury box. Then Judge Pratt entered. Everyone in the courtroom rose as the judge, impressive in his dark robe, crossed to the bench and seated himself.

With a sharp rap of a gavel, a court officer called for order. In the silence that followed he announced the case: United States of America versus Filipina Narciso and Leonora Perez.

Sitting with their lawyers, Perez and Narciso appeared calm and composed. Earlier that morning they had entered the courthouse, smiling at the cameramen gathered near the doors. Now they sat, attentive, as Judge Pratt began to speak.

Turning toward the jurors, he greeted them cordially. Then he explained that, although he had paraphrased the indictment against the defendants at the time of jury selection, he would now go into greater detail. He would read the indictment. Cautioning them that an indictment was but a formal means of informing them of the nature of the charges and should not be considered evidence, he continued, "Nor should any inference of guilt be made because these defendants have been charged in the indictment or because they are present here for trial." Then he began to read.

The first count in the indictment was the conspiracy charge, alleging that Narciso and Perez had knowingly, willfully, and unlawfully conspired to mingle poison in the intravenously administered food and medicine of patients at the US government's Ann Arbor VA hospital, with the intent to injure said patients. There followed a list of eleven overt acts charged against the defendants, the poisonings administered with the intent to injure and the murders undertaken with premeditation, deliberation, and malice aforethought.

The courtroom was silent as Judge Pratt read. Perez and Narciso sat, unmoving. When he had finished, Pratt set the indictment aside and turned to the jurors. "Now those are the counts of the indictment," he said, "which you must eventually determine."

Since many of the jurors were inexperienced, he would explain the trial procedure, he said. There would be opening statements from both the prosecution and the defense. There would be witness testimony and cross-examination of witnesses and finally closing statements by the attorneys. He spoke of the jurors' duty to weigh the evidence they would hear and draw reasonable inferences from that evidence. Then he paused. "[T]he right to a jury trial is a hollow right," he said, "unless all the jurors act intelligently, conscientiously and impartially. That involves, of course, your retaining your objectivity and not being swayed by sympathy, prejudice or any other emotion. The function of the jury is one that has been handed down to us for many centuries, and now you are cast in that role."

Then, turning, he said, "All right, Mr. Yanko, would you like to begin, please?"

Assistant US Attorney Richard Yanko, now head of the prosecution team, rose from his seat and walked to the podium where he would speak. He was a slender, dark-haired man of medium height wearing large, heavily framed eyeglasses that seemed to lend gravity to an otherwise youthful face. Spreading his notes on the podium, he introduced himself, the other attorneys for the prosecution, and the FBI agents who were sitting at the prosecutors' table. Then, looking at the jurors, he took a deep breath and began to speak.

"History, ladies and gentlemen, is in the making today in this courtroom, dark history, criminal history, history our ancestors never willed upon us, history which our descendants will look upon with disdain. We commence today to reveal events, sordid events, which ought never to have occurred. We begin today the task of analyzing a dreadful series of happenings which we will later seek to suppress and erase from our memories."

He continued, "Fourteen days in the heat of July and August, 1975; fourteen days, six of which must now be relived, days which produced eleven events which now comprise the subject matter of this trial."

Slowly he listed the eleven events, naming the patients who had been poisoned and those who had died, giving the time and place of each attack. Then he named the accused, saying, "Ladies and gentlemen, the last thing the United States desires in this case or in any case is for two innocent defendants to be found guilty or, if you turn that coin over on the other side, for two guilty defendants to be set free." The common goal, he said, was to determine the truth.

"As we now proceed, the eyes of the community are all upon us. In fact, the ears of the world will measure our every course. So then, let us begin our task. Let all men know that we seek not a prosecution at any price, but that we seek only one true goal, justice. Let all men know that we extend to these defendants the presumption of innocence and that we hallow that presumption."

Evidence about the crimes committed would emerge from witness testimony, he said. It was the jurors' duty to determine truth beyond a reasonable doubt. "However, if you believe for one minute that this case will present all black and white, forget it. If you think the testimony presented will create few problems, dismiss that thought also."

Proving that criminal acts had been performed would not be a simple task, he said. In preparing for the trial he had often thought it would be simpler to go a round with Muhammed Ali or wrestle a grizzly bear. They would hear vast amounts of complicated medical testimony. But, in fact, what the prosecution was trying to prove was simple: that somebody had injected a drug known as Pavulon into the IV tubing leading into the patients' veins, causing the patients to stop breathing; and that the injections were done secretly, without authorization, and with an intent to injure. "In a nutshell, ladies and gentlemen, that's what the testimony will prove."

"Now what testimony?," he asked. "What witnesses? The first witnesses you will hear will attempt to educate you in a general way, so that later testimony will be more understandable." Yanko went on to name some of these witnesses and to outline the testimony each would provide. "Then we will follow [with] an event-by-event recitation of the medical facts of each victim." This testimony would come from physicians assigned to the care of the patient and from doctors and nurses who had treated the patient at the time of his breathing arrest. Briefly he summarized the expected medical testimony for each of the events.

Then, leaning on the podium, he paused a moment, gazing at the jurors. "Now ladies and gentlemen, let us move to the ultimate question. What type of testimony will you hear?" He proceeded to tell them what they would *not* hear. None of the patients, not one, would say "I saw them do it. I saw Filipina Narciso and she had a syringe full of Pavulon. I saw her put that Pavulon into my intravenous tubing and she said, 'I want to hurt you.'" Nor would any witness claim to have heard either defendant expressing her intention to injure a patient. "That type of testimony is sometimes referred to as smoking gun testimony," Yanko said, "that is to say, a witness testifies, 'I saw the defendant leaving the scene of the crime with a smoking gun.' Well if we don't have that type of evidence, what do we have? We have the type of evidence which each one of us relies on every day, every hour. It's called inference. It's called logic. It's called reasoned conclusions. In the law we call it circumstantial evidence."

If a person were to enter the courtroom wearing a heavy overcoat and boots both covered with snow, Yanko said, it would be indirect evidence, circumstantial evidence, that snow was falling and the person had recently been outside in it. To have direct evidence of falling snow would require one to go outside and observe it. But such evidence was not available in this case. "Thus the evidence in this case will revolve around putting together various clues. The testimony offered will provide the clues," he said. And again Yanko summarized the expected testimony, making it clear in his summaries that at all eleven events of breathing failure one or both of the defendants had been present or nearby.

Earlier Yanko had declared that proof beyond a reasonable doubt did not mean truth beyond all doubt. Now he said, "At the conclusion of this trial, I am confident that you will find beyond any doubt whatsoever that eleven criminal acts were committed." And, more important, he said, they would find that Filipina Narciso and Leonora Perez had joined together in "a partnership of crime," conspiring to injure, poison, and murder helpless victims at the VA who had been entrusted to their care.

When reporters later asked Yanko why he had not addressed the question of motive in his statement, he said simply that motive was not essential to the government's case, but he added that if it were evident that the jurors were questioning what the motive might be, "We'd be prepared to answer."

CHAPTER 33

The following morning O'Brien stood before the jury ready to present his opening statement for the defense. Almost as soon as he began to speak it was apparent that his manner and tone were very different from Yanko's. Leaning easily against the podium, he introduced his client, Filipina Narciso. "You think maybe she wouldn't need to be introduced," he said, "but they ask for her pass every day when we come into court." The spectators chuckled. Every one of them had been required to show a pass to the federal marshals posted outside the courtroom doors in order to gain admission to the room.

O'Brien went on to introduce Ms. Perez and the other attorneys for the defense, Michael Moran, Edward Stein, and Laurence Burgess. Then he began his opening statement.

If Yanko's opening had been darkly dramatic, O'Brien's was low key, almost conversational. "There's a great deal you should know about this case," he said, "and a great deal you weren't told, and I knew I'd be standing here today to tell you. I think I'd like to begin with who the two people are that are on trial."

Both women had been born in the Philippines, he said. "You might think that they'd known each other before, that they knew each other in the Philippines, that their families had known one another all along. The truth of the matter is they met for the first time within weeks of the respiratory arrests in the summer of 1975."

Their lives were very different, he said, Ms. Narciso being single and Ms. Perez married and the mother of two. They had no social contact outside the hospital. In April 1975, Ms. Perez had transferred from the University of Michigan Hospital to the VA. In June 1975, only weeks before the respiratory arrests began to occur, the two had started work in the ICU. "Sometime in that month and a half, the government says, the great conspiracy was formed to commit the perfect crimes, to do what the government says you'll find no direct evidence of, only circumstances."

"Somehow, for some strange reason, two people who wouldn't have any reason in the world to harm patients, in a month, they claim, concocted this incredible scheme. That you will find to be nonsense. There wasn't any conspiracy between these two people. You wait for the day you hear the first witness get on that witness stand and say, 'I was there when they planned to kill patients.' Well, it isn't going to happen."

As O'Brien spoke, the broad outlines of the case for the defense began to emerge: the government had no direct evidence to offer, the tactics employed in the FBI questioning had been brutal, security at the VA was notoriously lax, any number of persons had access to patients, and the defense was prepared to name three others who had raised suspicions in this regard.

"We should talk a little about the VA hospital," O'Brien said. It was severely understaffed. Record keeping was "atrocious." As the defense attorneys tried to reconstruct what had happened, this fact had given them a great deal of trouble. There was no good record of who had been present at the arrests, no names. The response to Code calls was chaotic at best, and the events had been very poorly recorded.

The defense had monitored security in the ICU, he said, a place where one might expect careful watch to be kept on who came and went. "And do you know what? One hundred people, during one hour, during the monitoring time, came in and went out." The unit had automatic doors, he said, which opened like doors in a grocery store. You just stepped up to them and they opened.

"In other words what characterizes that hospital is there was an absolute lack of security. You could come and go at any time of the day or night without being stopped."

Now he moved on to the government's case. "The government was wise," he said, "when they told you they didn't have a smoking gun because there isn't one. They don't have any witnesses they can call who will say that these women injected patients for a very simple reason, they didn't.

"The defense is simple. The women didn't do the things they [the prosecutors] claim. And they said that from the beginning, and the FBI wouldn't listen and the FBI wouldn't believe them."

The FBI had had troubles that summer, O'Brien said. There were the unsolved Hoffa and Hearst investigations. There was a good deal of criticism of the bureau for other reasons. So, "a Federal hospital has a series of breathing arrests. Can't you imagine the word was, 'Get in there and find out what happened and solve it.'"

"[A]nd into the hospital they went. Within a couple of days, I think, they had a suspect. And what do you do when you have a suspect? Try to get them to confess—and, boy, did they try to get them to confess.

"What was done was shocking and revolting. It was a blatant violation of their rights. But they didn't confess."

He related that "on one occasion they had Miss Narciso in the hospital for six hours. She asked to go, and they wouldn't let her. They kept pounding. They wanted her to confess. And she said, 'I can't confess for things I didn't do.'"

O'Brien continued, speaking of the arrests that had occurred in the

ICU on the fifteenth of August: "[T]here are some things that you weren't told about that I think are vital for you to know." There was a nurse that Dr. Goodenday had seen standing beside Olson's bed as he was arresting. Dr. Goodenday had described that nurse's appearance in terms that did not fit Narciso. "Now, we will find out that there *are* a couple of people who match that description." One, he said, was a nursing aide who had been granted immunity by the government in exchange for grand jury testimony and who had been in the room with Olson all the time. "[T]he other was a nursing supervisor at the VA hospital who had some very serious problems." She had written a note declaring that the defendants were innocent. She had told a number of people, "You will be surprised to find out in the end who really did this." He spoke of the man in the green scrub suit that a patient had seen leaving his room just as his arrest began, a man observed in other places in the ICU during the period of arrests on the fifteenth.

"Well, the government was right," O'Brien said, "there won't be any direct testimony that these women injected anybody.

"Doesn't it seem reasonable that if these women, in fact, were walking around the hospital trying to kill patients, that somebody someplace would have seen them at a medicine chest, loading a syringe with Pavulon, that there would be a weapon somewhere, a syringe that was used, that there would be fingerprints on medical apparatus?

"You mean we're just all going to have to kind of infer that at the end we will take one circumstance and put another circumstance on top of it, and another and another and another, and try [to] somehow what? In your mind fill in what they can't do?"

The government's case was like a child's house of cards, O'Brien said, and like such a house it would not hold together. It would fall apart.

"I think, in the end, you will find that the defense will bring you closer to an understanding of what happened in the summer of 1975 than the government, with its millions of dollars and 200 FBI agents will do.

"And I think, in the end, we will all be able to go home, comfortable that justice was done and innocent people were not convicted."

O'Brien left the podium and walked back to the table where the other defense attorneys sat. Judge Pratt turned to them and spoke to Edward Stein, the attorney representing Leonora Perez. "Mr. Stein," he said, "your opening statement, please."

CHAPTER 34

Stein rose and walked quickly to the podium. He began at once. "What kind of place is the Ann Arbor Veterans Hospital? What kind of hospital is it where for three weeks patients stop breathing? What kind of place is it where that happened in the first place and where it continued for three weeks, until finally somebody decided to do something about it?"

Like O'Brien, Stein was a relatively young man, dark haired and sporting a neatly trimmed mustache, but his challenging opening announced a very different approach. Gone was O'Brien's low-key, conversational tone, his aim to "visit awhile" with the jury, as he had called it. Stein made no attempt to "visit." He launched directly into an attack on the hospital's administration.

"What kind of place is it where, when they decided to do something it included calling in the FBI, sending them running off in all direction without any medical training and without any training in hospital procedures and without any training in respiratory arrests, with the instruction 'solve our problem for us.' What kind of place is that?"

The VA was a kind of cousin, "perhaps a poor cousin," of the University of Michigan Medical Center, Stein said. While the affiliation was positive in many ways, it created problems with which the VA didn't deal. There was no permanent house staff. Residents not yet fully trained in their specialties and interns just graduated from medical school arrived at the VA, spent two or three months there, and were replaced with more new doctors who weren't familiar with the hospital or the patients and hardly knew one another. There were no security measures in place to deal with this situation, to make sure that the wrong people weren't treating the wrong patients at the wrong time with the wrong medications.

"In the summer of 1975 no one was in charge of the hospital," Stein said. The chief of staff was on leave for six months. For each of those six months a different doctor acted in his place. "[T]he bottom line is nobody was running the store and that's when the breathing arrests occurred."

Then he shrugged. "Well, I shouldn't say nobody was running the store because there was a committee. There's always a committee. And I guess they were running the hospital. And you'll hear about some of their meetings.

"You'll hear about those doctors and nurses who worked on the front lines and worked like they never worked before and saved lives, including Miss Narciso and Mrs. Perez.

"And they said to each other, 'What's going on here? What's happening?'

"And they said to their superiors, 'What's going on here? What's happening?' And their superiors reacted. They took it up at their committee meeting and they said, 'Well, the weather's hot, maybe that's the reason.'" Stein shrugged again and smiled a little, looking at the jurors.

"Finally they called in the FBI," he said, "and in came the FBI 'en masse.' Most of what the agents encountered was entirely unfamiliar, but they were under enormous pressure to solve the problem. They solved it by charging two of the evening shift nurses in the ICU.

"Well, it's simple and it's neat and it's tidy and it doesn't go any higher. And it's wrong and you'll know it when you hear the witnesses and the testimony.

"You won't hear about motive. Mr. Yanko talked for two hours and he couldn't give you a reason the government says these women went around trying to kill patients."

What would they hear? "Well, you are going to hear witnesses who have been hypnotized. That's right. The FBI hired some psychiatrist from New York, had him put these witnesses in a trance and then the FBI agents, who had already determined who the suspects were, went ahead and interrogated them [the patients] in an effort to firm up their case."

They would hear testimony about Pavulon, he said, about whether or not it had been found in the tissues of patients who had been exhumed, about the tests that had been devised to test for it. "[T]he FBI claims to have done what no university, no laboratory, no medical school in the world has done; found Pavulon in human tissue using the tests that they devised."

The government's case was circumstantial, he said, and circumstantial evidence had to be seen in context, kept in focus, or it was misleading. "You must keep each count in context—and keep it all in focus. By that I mean with respect to each count, each charge, looking at that as if it were the only charge before you.

"You can't take pieces from different counts and put them together, because they don't fit. You can't take pieces from different jigsaw puzzles and make a picture."

They would have to listen to the testimony and keep the context in focus. To do that would be very tough, very taxing, he said. "But that is what you have to do. —You know there is only one thing that stands between Filipina Narciso and Leonora Perez and their being convicted of crimes they did not commit—it is you. And let me tell you, by the time you have heard it all and you have seen it all you are going to have some help in the form of reasonable doubt.

"[F]inding reasonable doubt at the end of this trial will not be tough. You won't have to search for it, it's going to be all over the courtroom. It's going to surround you and it's going to scream at you and it's only screaming one message: Not guilty."

When Stein had finished, Judge Pratt suggested taking a short recess so that the jurors could "stretch a bit." Doubtless the jurors were glad to have the opportunity. The opening statements for the defense had consumed most of the morning.

CHAPTER 35

Assertions by the defense that there were other potential suspects in the case were duly reported in the press. Both the *Detroit Free Press* and the *New York Times* ran articles reporting that there were three other individuals under suspicion, including "a mysterious man in a surgeon's scrub suit" seen near patients who had been poisoned and a nursing assistant who had been granted immunity from prosecution. The *Free Press* quoted O'Brien as saying, "We'll hear an awful lot about her. Why she was granted immunity—what she did that she thought was criminal—will develop as the trial goes along."

Defense claims that the hospital lacked adequate security were also widely reported and seemed to be borne out in testimony given by the prosecution's first witness.

Gary Calhoun, assistant to the hospital's chief of the medical service, took the witness stand and was sworn in late Tuesday morning, following the jury's brief recess. Calhoun had been called by the prosecution to provide testimony that would "educate the jury" as Yanko had promised in his opening statement. He was to explain the organization of the hospital and its general operating procedures.

In response to Yanko's questions, he spoke at length, leaning forward and frowning with concentration as he described in detail the functioning of the hospital. Calhoun was a dark-haired young man who spoke with an appealing candor. He seemed determined to reply to Yanko's questions with as much information as he possessed.

When he turned to the subject of nurses, he admitted that there was a shortage. There were fewer employees to care for patients at the VA than at other hospitals in the area, he said.

"Had this caused difficulties in terms of overworked staff?," Yanko asked. Calhoun admitted that it had and spoke of the petition signed by a group of nurses that expressed dissatisfaction with their working conditions. Already he had testified that there were times when an RN might be covering two or three wards, moving from floor to floor and leaving some areas without another RN in her absence.

When attorney Burgess began his cross-examination he took up the question of security. He asked about persons who came and went every day in the hospital: volunteers, dieticians, technicians, delivery people, and maintenance staff. They could come and go pretty much as they pleased?, he asked. Calhoun agreed that they could.

"What about visitors to the hospital?," Burgess asked.

In the ICU the hours were rigid, Calhoun said. "But for the general hospital it is pretty much up to the nursing supervisor on the ward."

"Assuming she's there, of course, on the floor," Burgess said drily.

Still referring to the summer of 1975, Burgess said, "Let's assume you have a person that comes before the end of visiting hours. What would they do if they came into the hospital? Would they just walk over to the elevators and go up to the floor?"

"Probably."

"Probably? No sign-in procedure?"

"No."

"No passes?"

"No."

"So anyone could come and go in that hospital and go to any one of the floors we are talking about between the hours of—what in the morning?"

"I believe it is nine. I believe it is nine to nine."

"For a 12-hour period, nine to nine—anyone from the outside could come and go in that hospital without ever having to sign in, get a pass or anything else is that correct?"

"Yes, sir."

Burgess asked whether in 1975 there had been a way to identify an employee coming in after duty hours.

There was no badge or anything like that, Calhoun said, but there were employee ID cards. If the hospital security guard was there beside the elevators when an employee came in after duty hours, he would ask for an ID card.

"You are saying *if* he was there?"

Calhoun explained that the policeman made rounds throughout the hospital and its outer buildings. He might not always be beside the elevators. "So, during the time he is making rounds, anybody who came in—could go up the elevators to whatever floor they want."

Calhoun nodded. "Could."

At the back of the courtroom, reporters scribbled rapidly. It seemed certain that the lapses in security that Calhoun had mentioned would be noted on front pages the next day.

The following morning when attorney Michael Moran continued the cross-examination, he raised questions about a policy in the hospital that involved periodically locking psychiatric patients out of their rooms. Calhoun explained that the policy was part of the patients' treatment. Most were paranoid schizophrenics, he said. They typically withdrew from activities and secluded themselves. To keep them out of their rooms was a way to prevent such withdrawal.

They could mingle freely in the hospital?, Moran asked. They could not, Calhoun replied. They were on locked wards.

"Are you aware of the hospital practice of housing them elsewhere, other than on the 7th and 8th [psychiatric] floors?," Moran asked.

If a patient with a psychiatric disorder had a disease or injury necessitating his being placed on a surgical or medical ward, he would be on that ward, Calhoun replied.

And, Moran asked, would there be special measures taken to prohibit the patient from mingling with others in the hospital?

"Not routinely."

Moran had a reason for concentrating his questions on psychiatric patients. During the summer of 1975 such a patient, who was being treated for a medical problem on the fifth floor, had been discovered wandering in a room on that floor where a patient had undergone an arrest. Significantly, this patient was listed in the indictment as a victim of murder.

CHAPTER 36

On Tuesday, during a recess in the proceedings, a large, draped object some five or six feet long was wheeled into the courtroom, mounted on a rolling table. The spectators craned to look, but whatever lay beneath the drapery was entirely hidden from view. Wednesday morning the table still stood against a wall in the courtroom, its burden still covered. As Gary Calhoun's testimony continued, the spectators eyed the mysterious object with growing curiosity, speculating on what might be concealed beneath the heavy cloth.

It was midmorning before the attorneys declared that they had no further questions for Calhoun. Judge Pratt announced that there would be a recess, and, standing and stretching, the jurors left the courtroom. When they returned a short time later, attorney Yanko called the next witness for the prosecution.

A small, balding, bespectacled man rose from his seat and crossed the room to settle in the witness chair. His name was Raymond Schaeffer, he said. He was a visual information specialist with the FBI in Washington, DC, employed making charts and diagrams and models that were used to impart information in various ways. He had been doing this for twenty years.

"Were you requested to do any particular work for this particular case?," Yanko asked.

Schaeffer nodded. "Yes sir. I was requested to go to Ann Arbor to the Veterans Hospital and make a model of the East wing, third floor." That would be the Intensive and Coronary Care Units, he explained.

"Do you see the model in the courtroom today?," Yanko asked.

Schaeffer smiled proudly. "Yes, sir. Right there." He nodded toward the draped table.

Yanko asked him to step down from the stand and approach the table. The *Ann Arbor News* reported that Schaeffer was like "one of those kindly old cobblers you find in fairy tales" as, stepping down from the stand, he crossed the room and, "beaming with unabashed pride of accomplishment," grandly unveiled his creation.

He and two others had spent eight months constructing the model, he said, using photographs, diagrams, and measurements he had made on a visit to Ann Arbor in May 1976. Three-quarters of an inch represented one foot. "And I'd say she's accurate within half an inch in any direction," Schaeffer said.

The model, Government Exhibit Number Three, was intended to help jurors visualize the ICU and the complicated comings and goings there as the arrests were occurring. Yanko asked to have the table wheeled toward them and tilted to afford a better view. The jurors leaned forward eagerly.

What they saw was a miniature ICU, complete in every detail. There were eleven tiny beds, each supplied with a miniscule tray table and a heart monitor several sizes smaller than a postage stamp. There were miniature sinks fashioned of plastic, medicine cabinets, trash cans, laundry carts, and telephones, all rendered to scale. Curtains could be opened and closed at each window. Privacy curtains hung beside each bed on racks no bigger than toothpicks. Inhabiting this lilliputian world were plastic figures that had been modeled in conformity with dimensions supplied by the Bureau of Statistics, Schaeffer said. They represented adults of average size.

The jurors seemed fascinated. Even the defense attorneys looked bemused as they gazed at the model. But when they began their questioning their tone was challenging. O'Brien asked whether the diagrams Schaeffer had made in 1976 accurately reflected the unit as it had been in 1975. He asked how much the model had cost the government. Schaeffer seemed taken aback by this question. He had no cost analysis, he said. The cost was figured into the budget.

The *Detroit Free Press* later described the model as "a cross between a child's dream and a chamber of horrors." Beguiling as it was in all its tiny detail, it was, of course, intended to represent the site of several attempted murders, and, although Raymond Schaeffer might bring to mind the kindly cobbler in a fairy tale, his creation evoked associations far removed from a children's story.

* * *

Thursday morning the prosecution called Timothy Wiley to testify. Wiley, who had been assistant chief pharmacist at the VA in 1975, was a soft-spoken man with the earnest manner of an Eagle Scout. In response to the attorney's initial questions, he frowned in concentration.

He described his duties and functions as a pharmacist and then the procedures followed in the pharmacy for dispensing drugs. As he described them, the procedures seemed clear and straightforward. Drug orders came to the pharmacy, often by pneumatic tube. They were signed by the ordering physician or an RN. The pharmacist or technician who filled the prescription signed as well, and another signature was required from the person who picked up the medication at the pharmacy or received it if it was delivered to the floor.

Wiley explained the procedures in detail, giving a picture of a well-controlled system, but when Laurence Burgess began his cross-examination Wiley acknowledged that not all procedures were rigorously followed. Further, he acknowledged that once a bag filled with a prescribed medication left the pharmacy to be delivered elsewhere in the hospital it was possible that tampering could occur.

He agreed that en route or after they had reached the floor where they were needed these small, plastic "piggyback bags," as they were called, could be adulterated. It was conceivable, he said, that someone could inject a substance into a bag so that it would mingle with the prescribed medication. When the bag was later connected to a port in a patient's IV tubing, the unauthorized substance would flow into the patient's bloodstream together with the fluid dripping from the primary IV. Wiley seemed to recoil from the possibility, but he admitted it could happen.

Burgess pushed on with his examination. "Did there come a time when you did an inventory in the pharmacy to determine how much Pavulon was stored and used?," he asked.

Wiley hesitated. "We did an inventory. I believe, on or right after the 15th [in 1975]," he said. The inventory had revealed that twenty-five glass ampules of Pavulon were missing and could not be accounted for. Contained in the missing ampules was enough drug to paralyze some two hundred patients. The following day two empty ampules of Pavulon were discovered on the fifth floor, and Wiley could not account for this either. Pavulon was not used on the fifth floor. The pharmacy had not delivered it there. But, as the jurors would learn in the coming days, two arrests had occurred on the fifth floor on the fifteenth of August, one resulting in death.

The disappearance of the ampules was a startling revelation. To the jurors, it must have seemed bizarre. Wiley had already testified that Pavulon was stored and available in several locations in the hospital. Why would a person wanting to obtain the drug for an illicit purpose risk stealing twenty-five ampules from the pharmacy when it could easily be obtained at a number of other locations? Wiley had no explanation.

As O'Brien had said in his opening statement, the attorneys for the defense were under no obligation to prove anything. Rather, their task was to sow doubt and provoke questions about the evidence the prosecution offered. It seemed that in cross-examining Wiley and Calhoun they had made some progress. From both witnesses they had elicited testimony that seemed to support the contention that questionable security arrangements and procedures in the hospital in 1975 had offered ample opportunity to any number of people who might have wished to obtain Pavulon and gain access to patients.

CHAPTER 37

On Monday morning Dr. Marcelle Willock was seated on the witness stand. Willock was an anesthesiologist at Roosevelt Hospital in Manhattan and a consultant to the chief medical examiner in New York City. An attractive African American woman, she was an acknowledged authority in the field of anesthesiology. She had come to Detroit to serve as an expert witness for the prosecution.

Already she had testified at length about the use of muscle relaxants in operating rooms and ICUs. She had testified to the effects observed when various muscle relaxants were injected into the bloodstream and had spoken of the ways the drugs could be introduced into an IV apparatus. Now she was prepared to demonstrate some of what she had described. Rising from the witness chair, she went to stand before the jury.

The prosecutors had arranged an exhibit to facilitate the demonstration. Suspended from what appeared to be a coatrack were two large, plastic IV bags, each connected to a long slither of plastic tubing. Attorney Delonis asked Willock to point out various features of the model that she had mentioned in her testimony.

Accordingly, speaking to the jurors, Dr. Willock pointed out the clamp on the model that could be adjusted to control the speed of the IV flow. She indicated three sites where a drug could be injected directly into the tubing attached by a needle to a patient's vein.

Now Delonis handed her a syringe filled with blue dye and asked her to make an injection into one of these sites. Willock took the syringe and pushed the plunger. The blue fluid took only seconds to course down the tubing and empty into a wastebasket positioned to receive it. "[A]t this point it's already in the patient's bloodstream," she said.

She repeated the procedure, injecting a second site with similar swift results. A bolus, or rapid-push, injection at one of these sites was the usual way to administer a muscle relaxant, she said, the objective being to obtain rapid results in either the operating room or intensive care.

"[I]f somebody wanted to give a medication by putting it in the large bag," Delonis asked, "could that be done with a syringe?"

It could, Dr. Willock said, but you would do that only if you wanted to dilute the medication and give it over a longer period time, over perhaps eight hours. A bolus injection into the other sites would be in a patient's bloodstream in seconds. Half a minute later the effects of the drug would be observable.

Because the head and neck receive the largest blood supply, she said, the effects would be apparent there first. The patient's vision would blur. His eyelids would grow heavy. He would have a choking sensation as his tongue fell back into his throat, and then, quickly, he would begin to lose the ability to move his arms and legs. Failure to breathe would come last as the diaphragm became paralyzed, but it would occur in two or three minutes. If a large dose were injected, the entire process might take only sixty seconds.

"But if you took the same quantity," Delonis asked, "and were to place it in the bag itself and then set the bag at a normal drip rate over the period of eight hours, would you get the kind of effect you wanted from the drug?"

Willock shook her head. "Probably not," she said. The drug would be so diluted in the IV fluid and would enter the patient's bloodstream in such minute amounts over that period of time that the effects would be very slow to appear or might not appear at all. The patient might experience some blurred vision, but he would have time to call for help, unlike a patient who had received a bolus injection.

This testimony was of extreme importance to the prosecution. The symptoms displayed by the patients listed in the indictment appeared consistent in every case with those Dr. Willock described as typical of a rapid, or bolus, injection. The few seconds elapsing between such an injection and the onset of its effects would mean that whoever had given the injection would almost certainly still be nearby, would not have had time to go far, and would likely have been observed in the vicinity. The prosecution's case rested on the forthcoming testimony of witnesses who had observed Perez or Narciso, or both, in the vicinity of most of the 1975 arrests.

* * *

When he began his cross-examination of the witness, attorney Stein was quick to return to the subject of the large, or primary, IV bags, establishing that Dr. Willock had no personal experience administering muscle relaxants from these bags and had read little about the effects of the drug if it were administered in this manner. Now, holding up a glass ampule, Stein asked, "[T]he Pavulon in this clear ampule is also clear, is it not?"

"Yes, it is."

"And if this Pavulon were injected into this bag or this bag," he said, indicating the IV bags suspended from the coatrack, "there's no way we could tell that by looking at the bags?"

"Correct."

"Now, the testimony has also been, Dr. Willock, —that when these [indicating the small piggyback bags that would contain medications ordered for patients] are brought up to the floor from the pharmacy, they are put down in the ICU on a counter, and either they stay there or in an unlocked refrigerator or near the patient's bedside until they are ready to be used. And then the nurse responsible for giving the medication picks up the bag, hangs it and connects it to the tubing. Okay?"

"Yes."

"Now, if while that bag was sitting there and somebody injected 5 cc's of Pavulon into it, and then walked away and the bag remained there, and hours later a nurse picked it up to give medication, she wouldn't be able to tell there was Pavulon in it, would she?"

"No."

"And if she hung it and connected it and started the drip, the patient would be getting Pavulon, right?"

Dr. Willock nodded. "Yes."

"And the person who put Pavulon into the bag wouldn't even have to be in the hospital when it was given to the patient, isn't that correct?"

Dr. Willock agreed that it was.

Later, responding to Delonis's redirect examination, Dr. Willock testified that Pavulon, unrefrigerated and left on a counter or at a patient's bedside, would, in a warm room, lose some of its potency. And again there was the question of dilution. She believed that the drug could also lose potency if it remained in solution, as in a piggyback, for a period of time.

The next day a half dozen newspapers reported these qualifications but focused chiefly on Willock's agreement with Stein's hypothetical scenario. That someone could inject Pavulon in the manner he suggested and be far from the scene when the patient received the drug opened the door to myriad possibilities. The *Detroit News* termed a bag so injected "a medical 'time bomb.'"

"In my view Marcelle Willock was excellent, with a clear exposition of the facts. The cross-examination by Mr. Stein was, I felt, a valiant attempt but not very effective. I believe Dick Yanko felt otherwise, felt that the cross-examination by Stein was devastating. I clearly disagree." These observations are Dr. Martin Lindenauer's, contained in an ongoing record he was keeping of each day's trial proceedings. As chief of staff at the VA, he was, of course, deeply concerned with the progress in the case and clearly smarting from the highly critical view of the hospital administration expressed both by the defense and repeatedly in the media. Daily he drove from Ann Arbor to Detroit to be present in the courtroom. On the return trip he dictated his observations into a tape recorder.

On this April afternoon his comments concerned an argument he and Agent Russo had had with Yanko about the "time bomb" theory. "Yanko pursued in an aggressive way the possibility that there could be a 'time bomb' effect or way of administering Pavulon. There ensued a very difficult, heated argument with Russo walking out of the room and my shouting at Yanko."

Lindenauer and Russo were maintaining that Stein's theory that there could have been a delayed reaction to the drug was only that, a hypothesis advanced to weaken the prosecution's argument for bolus injections. But Yanko *had* to consider it as a possibility. Willock herself had agreed that such a means of administering Pavulon was possible. Although in response to redirect questioning she had said that dilution in an IV bag would diminish the drug's potency, Yanko could not ignore the fact that his own witness had agreed with Stein's proposed scenario.

"Subsequent to this meeting there was a good deal of bad blood between Russo and Yanko. For a day or two they were not talking to each other," Lindenauer recorded. "Later I called Yanko. I told him he was foolish, that this was a long, hard trial, that he had to depend on others and he had to exhibit faith in their ability and knowledge. —He took it well and promised to try to work together with everyone, so the team got together again." But clearly the stress of the trial had begun to take its toll.

CHAPTER 38

Of the eleven patients listed in the grand jury indictment, five had been receiving piggyback IV medications on the days of their arrests. At any rate they should have been. The medications had been ordered. The pharmacy had filled the bags and delivered them to the floors where they were needed to be administered at prescribed four- or six-hour intervals. But whether or not the medications *had* been administered as ordered was in question.

Byron Opstad, chief pharmacist at the Ann Arbor VA, had been called by the prosecution to testify regarding the solutions the eleven patients had been receiving just prior to their arrests. Opstad spoke carefully, precisely. He had done an exhaustive review of the patients' charts he said, producing a sworn statement listing the solutions each was scheduled to receive.

All eleven had been receiving nutrients in solutions flowing from the 1,000 cc primary bags hung on racks beside their beds. In addition, several were to receive antibiotics administered in piggyback solutions. Typically, the pharmacy prepared and delivered a twenty-four-hour supply of bags to be administered at the intervals prescribed, Opstad said. But, as he testified during cross-examination, in his review he had found that several charts lacked any notation indicating that the medications had been administered.

Such documentation should have been there, he said. Correct procedure required an initialed notation in the chart, confirming that the medication had been given as ordered. But in several of the charts he reviewed he had found no such notation.

So either the medications were not charted or were never given?, attorney Stein asked. The Joint Commission for Accreditation of Hospitals considered a dose not recorded as not given, Opstad replied.

Of course it was possible that an overworked nurse with an overload of patients might forget to record a medication she had given and improbable that a physician's order had been intentionally disregarded. But, as with other testimony already elicited in cross-examination, Opstad's report of this absence again raised questions about hospital practices.

His testimony may also have lent some weight to the "time bomb" idea. Had someone wanted to inject a bag with Pavulon, the pharmacy's customary delivery of bags in twenty-four-hour supplies would have provided a number of bags to choose from and considerable time for the undertaking.

Stein had no further questions. Opstad stepped down from the stand. In the stuffy courtroom there was an almost palpable sense of weariness. It was Friday. The week of proceedings was drawing to an end. The jurors seemed restless as they waited for the judge to excuse them for the weekend. The attorneys had begun stowing papers into their briefcases. When Judge Pratt announced the adjournment that afternoon, the courtroom emptied rapidly.

The following Monday the prosecutors asked to have six photographs entered into evidence. Of the six, three were photographs of primary 1000 cc bags containing IV solutions; the others were photographs of bags containing urine samples. This was the collection that had been retrieved from patients arresting on the fifteenth of August, ordered collected by Dr. Anne Hill. For seventeen months the bags had been stored in a locked freezer at the US Food and Drug Administration (FDA) laboratory in Detroit.

Earlier in the trial John Wiley, the Chief Sample Custodian at the FDA, had brought the bags themselves into the courtroom packed in dry ice and had testified to the security measures taken at the FDA laboratory to ensure that there was no tampering.

Drs. Hill, Goodenday, and Bishop had already testified regarding their roles in the collection and securing of the IV solutions and urine samples on the afternoon of the arrests. Assistant Pharmacist Timothy Williams had testified that he had received the material in Dr. Bishop's office on the night of the fifteenth and taken it to a laboratory at the University of Michigan Medical Center the same night. There, according to two university pharmacists, it had remained in locked refrigeration with only small samples withdrawn for testing until Timothy Williams collected the material again and transported it to the FDA laboratory for further testing.

Establishing this chain of custody was an important first step in offering the photographs into evidence. The chain was meant to confirm that the material had been safeguarded and was never unaccounted for in the nearly two years since its initial collection.

In stating the prosecution's request that the photographs the specimens be admitted, attorney Westbrook summed up the testimony that had been offered to establish the chain. Turning to Judge Pratt, he said, "Your Honor, I would close simply by saying that we are required by law only to show that by reasonable probability there was no unauthorized tampering with the samples and that, in short, circumstantially the integrity of the chain was kept throughout."

As soon as Westbrook finished speaking, defense attorney Stein objected. "We very strongly object to the introduction of the proposed exhibits in question," he said, "not merely because there are gaps in the chain but because the chain never started." The government was asking the court to assume that the IV bags offered into evidence were the ones in place at the time of the arrests, he said, and that certain urine specimens had been taken from patients within the two-hour time period that Dr. Willock had described as critical for urine testing.

The government was going to claim that some of the urine had tested positive for Pavulon, he said. But of equal importance was the fact that the solutions in the IV bags had tested negative for the drug. This critical finding, he said, required reasonable certainty that the bags were in fact the ones that were in use at the time of the arrests. Although the bags were labeled for those particular patients, there was no indication that they had been administered at a given point in time.

This argument was important to the defense, which wanted to claim, despite Dr. Willock's earlier testimony, that the Pavulon could have been administered to the arresting patients through the primary IV bags over a period of several hours. This would do much to undermine the prosecution's insistence on bolus injections and the circumstantial evidence implicating Perez and Narciso in the arrests. The absence of Pavulon in the bags being offered as evidence would obviously destroy that argument. If, however, it could be argued that these were not the bags in use at the time of the arrests, the claim remained viable.

The next day Judge Pratt ruled that the photographs of the urine samples would be admitted into evidence, but he refused to admit photographs of two of the three primary bags, saying much what Stein had: although the bags were labeled as intended for specific patients, there was no indication that they were being administered at the time of the arrests. He agreed to admit the third bag containing Jordan Olson's IV solution. Dr.

Goodenday, who had been with Olson throughout his arrest, had taken down and secured his IV bag herself and could attest to its authenticity. No such authentication was available for the other bags.

★ ★ ★

In the trial's early days Judge Pratt had seen to it that the jurors were provided with notebooks. A good deal of the testimony they were to hear, he said, would be technical, complicated, and not always easy to understand. Taking notes about what they heard might help them in their later deliberations. When Milda Walters began her testimony late in the trial's third week, it seems likely that note taking was copious.

Walters, an analytical chemist at the FDA laboratory in Detroit, had been called as an expert witness by the prosecution. She was to testify about the analytic work she had done testing for Pavulon in the material just received into evidence, the three urine samples and Olson's IV solution.

What followed was a lengthy and complicated explanation of the testing she had done on Olson's solution. Her test results were negative, she said. She had detected no pancuronium, not one milligram in the thousand-milliliter solution. The results reported by a second analytic chemist from the FDA, who had done chromatographic work on Walters's extraction from Olson's solution, were the same: no Pavulon detected.

Evidently the chemists had similar testimony to offer about the contents of the other IV bags, testimony that could have added weight to the prosecution's argument for bolus injections. But they could not provide that testimony since the bags in question were not in evidence.

The day after the chemists' appearance, Yanko petitioned the court for permission to reopen the question of the bags' admissibility.

Citing legal precedents for such a reconsideration, he continued, calling the bags critical evidence. He admitted that the prosecution had not met the required standard of authenticity but said that the attorneys had had adequate reason to believe that the solutions were in fact the ones the arresting patients had been receiving.

Now the prosecution was prepared to call two witnesses—nurses who could provide testimony that the solutions being offered as evidence were those being administered to patients during the day in question.

The defense objected. It seemed that the prosecution hadn't thought about determining authenticity until it lost the attempt to have the evidence admitted, Attorney Moran declared. Attorney Stein argued that Narciso and Perez had the right to a speedy trial and reopening the question would result in further delays. "The Government seems to take the position that it is entitled to try as many times as it has to before it gets it right," he said. "Well, this isn't a legal seminar or spring training; it is a very important case; they are trying to send two people to prison and it's no place for Mulligans."

After Yanko spoke again at some length, Judge Pratt said he would take the issue under advisement.

On Monday morning, before the jurors entered the courtroom, Pratt announced his decision. He denied the government's request to reopen the question of the rejected bags. The government's arguments for reconsideration were not sufficiently persuasive, he said. His original ruling would stand.

The prosecutors' frustration was evident. According to sources, they had felt for some time that Judge Pratt's sympathies lay with the defense, and this ruling can only have intensified that feeling. It deprived them of evidence that would have added significant weight to their argument for bolus injections, and it left the defense argument intact.

CHAPTER 39

On the April 18, 1977, the fourth week of the trial began. The excitement surrounding the first weeks of the proceedings had begun to dwindle. The number of spectators had dwindled as well. Now, on most days, there were only twenty-five or thirty spectators in the courtroom and as few as six or eight members of the press. The television crews that had seemed permanently in place when the trial began were no longer there to greet the defendants when they arrived each morning.

The proceedings had begun to seem slow moving and tedious. Long descriptions of hospital procedures and chemical analyses, important as they were to the case, did not make for riveting news stories. But now the prosecution was expected to begin calling witnesses who had been involved in the events as they were occurring, and the reporters hoped this testimony would be more promising.

The first of these witnesses was a pleasant-looking, gray-haired woman who seemed anxious as she took the stand, glancing about uncertainly as Yanko stepped forward to begin his examination. Her name was Hannah Wiley, she said. She was familiar with the VA hospital because her husband George had been a patient there. In fact, he had died there, having suffered a stroke some weeks after experiencing two breathing arrests.

She had visited her husband every day, she said, staying from morning until late in the evening, and she was familiar with many of the doctors and nurses. In reply to Yanko's question, she identified Narciso as one of those nurses. "P.I." she called her, nodding toward the defense table. "She's right over there. The lady in green."

The prosecution had called Mrs. Wiley to testify about the arrest that Leonard Meadows had undergone on July 27, 1975. Now Yanko asked if she had had occasion to observe his problem. "Yes, I did," she answered. "I had been late on a Sunday afternoon in the ICU." The unit was unusually quiet, and there were hardly any visitors. She and her sister, Marilyn Gibson, had been standing at her husband's bedside, which was close to the bed where Mr. Meadows lay resting. She was talking with her husband, she said, when P.I. appeared and began talking with her sister. "I don't know where she come from. She just seemed to come up all of a sudden, and she said hello to my sister." P.I. had stayed only a few minutes before she left again, said Mrs. Wiley. "I didn't pay any attention to where she went."

"Then what happened?," Yanko asked.

Mrs. Wiley frowned. "Well, my sister said, 'Oh my God, Hannah, look at that man over there' and she was referring to Mr. Meadows, and he was throwing his arms and legs around and kind of short of breath. . . . So I said, 'Oh my God, I'd better get someone.'"

"I looked at the nurses' station, wasn't anybody there, so I run back in the corridor to where you go into the heart patients' area. . . . I said, 'Hey, somebody!' and I didn't see anybody." She saw nobody until she came to the medical supply room. There she saw a nurse, one she did not know or recognize. "And I yelled in there at her and she come out and we both ran back."

"How much time went by between the visit of Miss Narciso and the problem with Mr. Meadows?," Yanko asked.

Mrs. Wiley didn't know. She recalled only that Narciso had stood for a moment at the foot of her husband's bed, talking with her sister. She did not see Narciso again. She did not see Narciso approach Meadows's bed or go near him, she said.

As her testimony continued, Mrs. Wiley's confusion about events became apparent. She had told the FBI agents a different story when they originally questioned her, Yanko reminded her. "Well, when I was first questioned," she said, "I was telling them about another man I got help for and I hadn't thought about Mr. Meadows." In fact she hadn't thought about him until weeks later when her sister reminded her of the incident. "And I said, 'Oh my Lord,' I had completely forgotten about going for somebody for him."

As Yanko had doubtless known it would be, Mrs. Wiley's confusion was immediately addressed when O'Brien began his cross-examination. Comparing her testimony on the stand to statements she had made earlier to the FBI agents, he called her attention to the discrepancies in the two accounts, pointing out that she had mistaken one patient's emergency for another's, had in fact failed to remember Meadows's problem until reminded by her sister.

This victim-by-victim testimony was the bedrock of the prosecution's case. That Hannah Wiley had witnessed Leonard Meadows's arrest shortly after she had seen Narciso in the vicinity was the sort of circumstantial evidence on which the prosecution was depending. But there was enough confusion in Wiley's conflicting accounts to leave room for doubt about the dependability of her testimony.

When Mrs. Wiley's sister, Marilyn Gibson, testified next, she corroborated much of what Wiley had said about the events surrounding Meadows's arrest, but she did not agree with everything. When her sister returned from her search for help, Gibson said, the nurse with her was Narciso. Narciso was the nurse who hurried to hit the red alert button above Meadows's bed. Gibson referred to her as "Pia."

CHAPTER 40

When Bart Martin arrested in the CCU on July 29, 1975, Lula Balls was there. Balls was a plump, middle-aged African American woman, a nurses' assistant who was working in the ICU on the three-thirty to midnight shift. Of course she knew P.I. and Leonie, she told prosecuting attorney Westbrook.

She recalled that sometime between five and six on the twenty-ninth P.I. had come out of the CCU and asked her to watch Mr. Martin. P.I. wanted to get something to eat and asked Balls to keep an eye on him.

The CCU was quiet that evening, Balls remembered, no visitors around. Mr. Martin was the only patient in the unit. When she entered his room he was sitting up in bed eating supper. P.I. was standing at the foot of the bed.

Balls went over to the monitoring station to have a look at Martin's heart monitor, and so her back was turned. But she had heard P.I. speaking to him, telling him she was leaving the unit for a little while and she hoped he was enjoying his dinner. Soon after that P.I. left.

Mr. Martin lay back in bed like he was tired, Balls said. Then suddenly he reared back up again, went limp, and collapsed.

"From the time that Miss Narciso left the bedside to the time Mr. Martin sprang up and then down, how much time was that?," Westbrook asked.

"About five minutes."

"Could it be less than a minute?"

Balls shrugged. "It could be less."

Time was of course crucial to the prosecution's case. As Dr. Willock had demonstrated, Pavulon's effects would begin to be evident in less than a minute if given as a bolus injection in the IV tubing. It was important that Westbrook pin down the time frame as closely as he could.

He reminded Balls that she had made statements about time to the FBI agents when they questioned her and later in sworn testimony before the grand jury. In both she had said she thought only thirty seconds had elapsed between Miss Narciso's departure and Mr. Martin's collapse.

Balls looked rattled. Then she burst into tears. How could she know if it was thirty seconds or a minute?, she asked. "I was telling the truth as near as I could do it."

Later, on cross-examination, O'Brien asked her whether she had seen a syringe in Miss Narciso's hand and whether she had seen Miss Narciso bending over the patient's tray as he ate in order to administer an injection into his IV tubing.

Balls shook her head. "No," she said. She had seen nothing like that.

As would happen each time testimony was taken about a patient's arrest, physicians who had attended the patient testified at some length about the reasons for hospitalization and about the patient's condition prior to the arrest. Dr. Sadasivan had been questioned concerning Meadows. Now Dr. Roberta Kurtz spoke about Martin.

She had visited him on the afternoon preceding his arrest, she said. She had found him resting comfortably, with no complaints. Although he was being monitored for arrhythmia and evaluated for the insertion of a pacemaker, there was no indication that his heart had caused the arrest. The heart monitor showed no problems. "It was a respiratory arrest," she said. "He just couldn't breathe."

* * *

"Dictated today, returning back from a day in Detroit: Kurtz testified today and handled it just beautifully. She was convincing, forthright, sincere. She said that though Martin had some chronic illnesses, he was not acutely ill and his arrest was totally unexpected.

A few unkind cuts by Stein pointing out that on July 29 Kurtz had been a practicing physician for only 29 days. He also made a pitch about what I was doing there and my attempting to influence witnesses. Kurtz said that I had absolutely not influenced her in any way."

CHAPTER 41

The weather was unusually warm for late April. Judge Pratt's courtroom was hot despite the fans that were struggling to stir the sluggish air. Pratt apologized to the jurors for their discomfort and suggested that the attorneys might want to remove their jackets. At the back of the room the spectators sat, fanning themselves with handkerchiefs and magazines. But at the defense table Narciso and Perez sat, hands folded.

Early each weekday morning they were driven from Ann Arbor to Detroit to be present in court before 9:00 a.m. It had been nearly five weeks of early mornings now. Eventually they would testify in their own defense—attorney Stein had announced that to the press several days before the trial began—but so far they had only sat quietly, their composure seemingly undisturbed by the testimony they were hearing.

This morning they sat, watching, as an elderly man lowered himself slowly into the witness chair.

"Homer Mercer is the name," he said. "I'm in pretty fair shape considering my age. You know what I mean? You can't expect too much when you get old." Attorney Westbrook smiled. Homer Mercer was eighty-nine.

He had been hospitalized for bowel surgery. "That's the first operation I ever had," he said proudly.

"Now," said Westbrook, "do you recall at some point having a breathing problem at the hospital?"

Mr. Mercer shrugged. "[W]hen I was in Intensive Care for ten or twelve days, I didn't know where I really was or whether I was breathing or not."

In fact Mr. Mercer had experienced two breathing problems during his hospitalization. The evening following his operation he had the first one and was immediately placed on a ventilator. The next day, according to the testimony of his physicians, they had begun to "wean" him. That is, they had taken him off the ventilator for periods of time with apparent success. He had seemed to be breathing satisfactorily on his own. But that evening he underwent a second arrest.

His son, Robert, took the stand to describe the episode. He had spent a good deal of time in the ICU following his father's operation, he told attorney Yanko. On the twenty-ninth he left the unit long enough to have dinner. When he returned at eight-thirty or nine o'clock, he saw that his father was not on the ventilator. There was a nurse standing at the head of his father's bed, bending over and doing something with her hands, but her back was to him and he couldn't see what she was doing.

He had stood quietly at the foot of the bed. His father appeared to be sleeping. "And then I had a premonition that something was wrong," he said. "I was staring at him and I didn't see his chest moving. . . . [A]nd then all of a sudden, why he lifts up in bed. . . . It was almost like he was trying to scream, except there was no sound coming out." It was as if his father were trying to get air, Mercer said, like somebody hit in the diaphragm playing football.

"What did the nurse do?," Yanko asked.

"Just continued to look at him."

She made no movement, Mercer said. "And I screamed out, 'For Christ's sake, he's not breathing!' I yelled it very loud."

"When you yelled out, did the nurse do anything?"

"No." She didn't turn to look at him. She just stood there. But his yell brought a doctor and nurse running in from the corridor. They told him to leave the room.

In about fifteen minutes the doctor came out of the room and told Mr. Mercer that his father's condition was stable and he had been placed back on the ventilator. "He told me that he didn't give my dad much of a chance at all and that he had never seen somebody his age survive what he had gone through the night before. And he wanted to level with me and tell me straight out." Mercer was left with the impression that his father was dying.

He had been very angry about this episode. He seemed angry still as he related the events. He thought the nurse at the head of his father's bed was the same one who had suctioned his father's throat improperly on another day, not doing it the way the other nurses did. He had spoken to her about this. He had spoken to her supervisor.

"[D]o you feel you would still recognize her?," Yanko asked.

"Yes," Mercer said. "The gal in the red jacket."

"Let the record reflect that the witness has identified Leonora Perez," Yanko said, then asked if there was any particular characteristic about Ms. Perez that had enabled Mercer to make the identification.

"She has gold between two teeth," Mercer said.

He had seen the gold at other times when speaking with her. Months earlier he had been present at the lineup of nurses at the Westland police station, again recognizing Perez because of the gold in her teeth.

On cross-examination the defense returned to the gold. Mr. Mercer had testified, had he not, that the nurse at the head of his father's bed had never turned in his direction?

"That's correct."

How would he know that this nurse had gold in her teeth if she had never turned her head?, the attorney asked.

CHAPTER 42

"Monday. En route to Detroit. Over the weekend Yanko made a good release to the newspapers concerning the note he is attempting to get custody of. He said he thought it was a forgery."

Lindenauer was referring to the note Perez had obtained from Olson following his arrest, the note Narciso believed exonerated her in the matter, the note reading "If I see her again, I will not remember her." The prosecutors had a copy, but they wanted to look at the original.

In the absence of the jury, Yanko argued that Narciso's failure to provide the note to the FBI agents was irrational behavior if the note could serve to exonerate her. But if, in fact, it were a forgery, her refusal to produce it was understandable, as was the defense attorneys' failure to turn over the original. Yanko admitted that he had no evidence that the note was a forgery, but he wanted it evaluated. Judge Pratt ordered that a handwriting specialist be called to analyze the note after which he would rule on its admission into evidence. Clearly, if it were judged to be a forgery, it would give the prosecution strong evidence of conspiracy.

On this Monday morning, as the fifth week of the trial began, several nurses were called to testify about the arrests that had occurred on the thirtieth of July. For some time, of course, it had been clear that many of the VA nurses were angry with the hospital administration and hostile to the government's case.

One RN, testifying that morning, claimed that Dr. Lindenauer had ordered the FBI agents to limit their investigation to nurses. They were not to bother the doctors in the hospital, she said. Although later Lindenauer denied ever having issued such an order, the claim was duly reported by the media, indicating the hostility abroad in the hospital.

At midmorning Doris Clark took the stand. She was an RN, she said, and had been working part time in the ICU in the summer of 1975 on the same shift as P.I. and Leonie.

"Do you recall an evening when Miss Narciso and Mrs. Perez went to visit a patient in another area of the hospital?," Yanko asked.

Mrs. Clark remembered it well. It had been near the end of July, early evening. The patient, Chester Rice, had been a patient in the ICU before he was transferred to the fourth floor. P.I. and Leonie wanted to see how he was doing. "They invited me to go," Mrs. Clark said, but she had not gotten on well with Rice during his stay in the unit. "He didn't like me," she said. And so she told P.I. and Leonie to go without her.

"And then what happened?," Yanko asked.

Doris Clark frowned. "[T]hen I remember P.I. coming back, breathless. And she said, 'We found Mr. Rice and I need a cut-down tray,'" which, Mrs. Clark explained, is a sterile tray containing the equipment needed to start an IV injection.

P.I. told her they had found Mr. Rice on the floor, evidently in arrest, she continued. "And, you know, she was real excited and out of breath and she got the cut-down tray and then just went back to assist."

On cross-examination O'Brien elicited praise for the defendants. They were excellent nurses, Mrs. Clark said, extremely conscientious. She had never seen them mistreat a patient. In all, her testimony had done little to assist the prosecutors.

Next a nurses' assistant who had been working on 4West on the evening of Rice's arrest testified that one of her duties was to get whatever the nurses and doctors asked for during an emergency. "Why wouldn't a nurse go herself?," Yanko asked.

"Well, generally in an emergency the doctors and nurses are working on the patient."

"Now if you were on 4West and there were an emergency," Yanko asked, "and a cut-down tray was needed, where would you go?"

"To the utility room."

"And if there were none there?"

She would go to 4East or 5West, she said.

Why Narciso had run all the way back to the ICU to obtain a cut-down tray when there were others who could have gone and closer places to find one was puzzling and insufficiently explained, Yanko's questions implied. Was there some other reason that Narciso had left the Rice resuscitation?

* * *

Rice's Code had been called at 9:35. At 9:45 there was another on 5West. The nurse in charge of 5West that evening testified that the nurses' assistant on the floor had left to go to the emergency on the fourth floor and she had been alone with thirty-three patients to care for. "I was the only nurse on the floor," she said.

"[D]id you in fact discover the patient arresting?," Yanko asked.

"Yes. . . . Mr. Jackson was not breathing and he was pulseless."

She had headed for the nurses' desk to call a Code. In her notes in Jackson's chart she had recorded that she found him without a pulse and not breathing at 9:43.

Was it possible that in the ten minutes between Rice's arrest and Jackson's someone had had time to leave the one emergency and create another? It seemed that O'Brien was anticipating the question. He returned to a consideration of the numbers of persons who had easy access to patients that summer. Then he asked, hadn't it been only an hour before finding Jackson with no observable pulse that she had hung an IV piggyback bag for him?

"Yes," she said.

"Have you ever had the feeling that nurses in the hospital could innocently be hanging contaminated IV piggybacks?" he asked.

She had considered that, she said.

CHAPTER 43

Howard Jackson was pronounced dead at 10:30 on the night of the thirtieth. He had been a very sick man according to his physician's testimony. Seventy-four years old, a diabetic and an alcoholic, he had suffered from peripheral vascular disease resulting in the amputation of both legs several years earlier. He had gastrointestinal problems as well and had been admitted to the hospital vomiting blood. But it was a severe kidney infection that was his doctor's chief concern on the thirtieth. Jackson's temperature had risen to 104 degrees. The doctor had listed his condition as critical. Nevertheless, the doctor testified, he had not expected Jackson to die that day.

The severity of Jackson's condition was emphasized by the defense in cross-examining the doctor, the attorneys suggesting that the death of a man so very ill could be explained as the result of natural causes even though it not expected to occur so soon.

Already Mrs. Miranda Haber had testified to events on the evening of Jackson's arrest, and her testimony presented the defense with problems. Mrs. Haber was the widow of a patient who had occupied the room adjoining Jackson's on the night of the thirtieth. She had heard a lot of turmoil that evening sometime after nine o'clock, she said, with "all the commotion and machines down the hall and the nurses running and everything." She had heard banging in the room next door.

"And before the commotion, what was the ward like at that time?," Yanko asked.

"Very quiet."

"And how long did the commotion take place?"

"Probably twenty minutes to a half hour." In that half hour she had not left her husband's room but had sat on the windowsill from which position she could see into the corridor.

"Did there come a time on that particular evening that you were visited by nurses from other floors?," Yanko asked.

"Yes." Miss Narciso and Mrs. Perez had stopped by for a few minutes, Mrs. Haber said. She had gotten to know them when her husband was a patient in the ICU.

"When was this visit?"

"It was after the arrest." Everything had quieted down, she said. People were leaving.

So once again testimony placed the nurses near the scene of an arrest, but more important to the prosecution's case was confirmation that one or both had been in the vicinity *before* the arrest began.

"Now had you seen either of the nurses prior to that time?," Yanko asked.

"Yes." She had seen Miss Narciso pass by in the corridor some time before. Narciso had waved to her.

"And was she by herself?"

Again, "Yes."

Yanko asked how much time had passed between seeing Miss Narciso in the corridor and being visited by both nurses.

Mrs. Haber was vague. "A while between," she said.

"At the time you saw Miss Narciso in the hall, was it quiet?"

"It seemed to be. Yes."

"Were people moving equipment or machinery?"

"Not at that time."

Beginning his cross-examination, O'Brien established that Mrs. Haber's husband had died of cancer early the following morning. "Would I be right," he asked, "that, given the fact that this was such a serious and trying time for you and also that it's a considerable time now since the event, that you are not certain about the time between seeing Miss Narciso and the later visit?"

"Right."

Then O'Brien read aloud a portion of her interview with the FBI agents in which she reported having seen a Filipino nurse, alone, in the vicinity of Mr. Jackson's room but didn't remember if that was before or after the emergency. So at that time she hadn't been sure one way or the other, O'Brien suggested.

"Right," said Mrs. Haber. "Right."

* * *

Because of the questions surrounding his death, Jackson was one of the patients whose body had been exhumed to test his tissues for Pavulon. Lee Weatherbee, the VA pathologist who had taken tissue specimens from the body at the funeral home in October 1975 now testified, describing the procedure. The prosecution produced photographs of the specimens obtained and promised to establish a chain of custody before offering them into evidence.

Following Dr. Weatherbee, Roger Aaron took the stand. Aaron, a special agent for the FBI and a forensic chemist at its laboratories in Washington, had been present when Mr. Jackson's body was disinterred, he said. He had received specimens of tissue from Dr. Weatherbee enclosed in sealed plastic bags and had taken them to the FBI laboratories in Washington where they had remained in a locked freezer.

That much was simple and established a chain of custody. It was when Aaron began to describe the work he had done on the specimens from Jackson's liver and lung that his testimony grew complicated.

Although, as Milda Walters had testified, scientific literature existed concerning the detection of pancuronium in bodily fluids, there were no scientific reports about its detection in human tissue. In fact, Aaron knew of no one else who had done such work. In 1975, he said, Pavulon was a relatively new drug. It had been on the market for only about a year. "And it takes a long time for examination to be done on new products." It took a long time for papers and reports of results to appear in the scientific literature. "I had to develop a procedure myself," he said. For five months he had worked on developing this procedure.

"The majority of the problem was to do with the isolation and identification [of the drug]. After that the tests, themselves, were ones regularly used in drug analysis." Detecting the drug in embalmed tissue made the process at least ten times more difficult, he said, but he had devised a means of extracting the drug successfully from embalming fluid. Finally he was able to run tests on the specimens.

Before he could say much more, defense attorney Stein objected to the lack of scientific literature. "[B]y Mr. Aaron's own testimony," he said, "no one, apparently, except Mr. Aaron has ever claimed to have been able to extract Pavulon from human tissue."

In fact, Aaron had provided the defense with tissue samples and a detailed description of the procedure he employed to extract the drug so that an independent laboratory could repeat the procedure and confirm his findings. Apparently the defense had received a report from such a laboratory, but the attorneys chose not to mention it in court. Stein made a motion to exclude Aaron's testimony from evidence.

The next morning Judge Pratt denied Stein's motion, agreeing with the prosecution's argument. Although "no one has apparently tested for Pavulon in this way," he said, "that novelty does not in this Court's opinion require that the testing results and eventual opinion be held inadmissible."

Roger Aaron returned to the stand.

What followed was a lengthy, highly technical explanation of the work he had done on tissue specimens from Jackson's lung and liver.

Finally Yanko asked, "Mr. Aaron, in terms of the results of all these tests and extraction procedures—have you come to form an opinion as to the presence of pancuronium in Mr. Jackson's lung tissue?"

"Yes I have," Aaron said. "In my opinion pancuronium is definitely present in that lung tissue." It was definitely present in the liver tissue as well, he said.

Although Stein continued to ask questions designed to raise doubts about Aaron's methods and conclusions, the prosecutors had essentially won the day. And no doctor had ordered Pavulon for Howard Jackson.

CHAPTER 44

Nor had any doctor ordered Pavulon for Jeffrey Wallace. Yet on the evening of August 12 Wallace underwent a respiratory arrest, exhibiting all the symptoms that would later be recognized as typical of Pavulon poisoning.

Wallace was being treated for a fractured elbow. It was not a serious injury. The surgery to repair the fracture, undertaken at another hospital in the area, had been uncomplicated, "a minor operation," his physician called it. Transferred to the VA to recuperate, Wallace had been doing well. His physician expected him to be discharged from the hospital in a day or two. Then came the cardiac arrest.

Wallace had struck his head in the fall that fractured his elbow, but X rays taken at the VA at the time of his admission were inconclusive regarding a skull fracture. There was no evidence of brain injury, and a cardiac arrest accompanying a breathing problem was not unusual, his physician said. A breathing arrest could cause such a problem.

What *was* unusual was how quickly Wallace had responded to resuscitation. Although he was limp and unmoving following this procedure, within two hours he could open his eyes and squeeze the doctor's hand. His reflexes and mental state seemed normal. Overall, the physician said, he had seen no physiological reason for the arrest.

On cross-examination the defense attorneys sought to attribute the arrest to a concussion or other head injury, but when Wallace himself took the stand, he claimed that when he fell he had experienced none of the symptoms ordinarily associated with such injuries. He had never lost consciousness. In fact, he said, "I got up, got in the car, and drove down to the guy I was working for, and he took me to the hospital in Ypsilanti." Wallace recalled all the details.

But he had no recollection of what had happened to him on the night of his arrest. He could remember no one coming into his room after his wife left that evening. He guessed he had been dozing.

Wallace's arrest had followed another that evening, one that took place in an adjoining room. According to nurses' testimony, his had occurred no more than ten minutes after the first Code was called. As the Stross Committee report had noted, several of the arrests that summer had occurred in close proximity in terms of both time and location, as if the rush of activity surrounding the first had provided the opportunity for a second attack.

And there *had* been a good deal of activity at the first arrest a male nursing assistant testified. There had been lots of people coming and going. He remembered that Miss Narciso had been at the first Code. Mrs. Jakim had been there as well. But neither he nor the nurse managing the crash cart in the hall had seen anyone enter Wallace's room.

There was no testimony in the matter of Wallace that seemed to implicate Filipina Narciso in his arrest, nothing beyond her presence at the Code preceding his. Nobody had seen her near Wallace's room.

Two days later the pattern noted in the Stross report recurred. On the night of August 14 two patients arrested on 5West in rooms diagonally across the hall from one another. The first Code—Alex Brock's—preceded Douglas Berry's by less than fifteen minutes.

Filipina Narciso was on 5West that evening. She had been seen in the hall near the nurses' station early in the Brock Code, but the nurse who had seen her there could not remember her assisting at the resuscitation. A nurses' assistant had seen Narciso stepping off the elevator as the Brock Code began. And there was testimony that it was Narciso who discovered Berry arresting. Standing in his room, she had called out—"hollered," as one nurse put it—bringing help from a doctor attending Brock.

Yet the testimony concerning Filipina Narciso's whereabouts and activities on the night of the fourteenth was at best inconclusive. She had been on 5West. She had "hollered" an alert. But even this was contradicted by testimony from a nurses' assistant who had seen another woman, an African American nurses' assistant, enter Berry's room and emerge to declare that he was in trouble.

The defense was quick to establish that Betty Jakim had been at both arrests that night and that there had been many other people in the vicinity, fifteen or twenty milling around across the hall. The situation had been chaotic. It was hard to tell who was in charge several witnesses testified. There was no telling who might have slipped into Berry's room.

* * *

As Yanko said in his opening statement, the evidence presented by the prosecution would be strictly circumstantial in nature. There would be no smoking gun, no witness saying "I saw them do it," no patient claiming to have seen his attacker. As the trial moved into the sixth week this evidence had begun to seem less than compelling.

Testimony placed Filipina Narciso in the vicinity of five arrests, but only in the case of Bart Martin's had she been observed near the patient's bedside prior to the episode. And thus far the only testimony implicating Leonora Perez in *any* arrest had been that of Homer Mercer.

By now the jurors may have been wondering just how significant this testimony was. Where, after all, should the nurses have been if not attending to patients in the ICU and to emergencies on other floors? Could their mere presence be considered suspicious? It seemed that they were simply doing what, as RNs, they were expected to do. True, Mercer's testimony raised questions. It seemed to indicate that Perez had been slow or unwilling to recognize his father's emergency. But, outraged as he was, Mercer was not able to say that he had witnessed her doing anything to cause the problem. Nor could anyone say that Narciso had been observed doing anything suspicious with regard to Martin. Proximity appeared to be the only incriminating evidence being offered.

* * *

That Friday afternoon when the trial adjourned for the day, Judge Pratt announced that he was dismissing the jurors for a week's break. It may be that, knowing what lay ahead for them, he felt they needed a rest. When they returned, testimony would begin concerning the final arrests on August 15, the day on which five patients had stopped breathing in little more than an hour and Dr. Anne Hill's tests had raised the specter of

Pavulon poisoning. The testimony was expected to last from three to four weeks with as many as forty witnesses called by the prosecution. Following this, the defense would begin its presentation, which was expected to last another month. In all, it appeared that it would be at least July before Judge Pratt delivered his final instructions to the jury, and there was no knowing how long it would take the jurors to reach a verdict. The summer might come to an end before the trial did, people said.

CHAPTER 45

When the jurors entered the courthouse on the Monday following their break, they were leaving a sunny May morning behind. Whatever they had done during their week of freedom, they agreed that a week had not been enough to catch up on half the things they had left undone while they sat day after day in the jury box. They chatted, waiting to be called back into the courtroom where the everyday world would soon seem as distant as the bright May morning.

That day the testimony began, as Judge Pratt had known it would, with the events of August 15, 1975. On the fifteenth, in the late afternoon, three patients had arrested in the ICU within fifteen minutes. Arthur Lenz's arrest was the first to occur, and his widow was one of the first witnesses to testify when the trial resumed.

Holly Lenz looked nervous as she took the witness stand and admitted that she was when Yanko began his questioning. On the afternoon of August 15 she and her husband's sister had been together in her husband's room, she said. His sister had been bathing a rash on his legs to relieve a burning sensation he was complaining of. A "little nurse" had been there, too, untangling his IV tubing.

The nurse had come into the room to tell Mrs. Lenz and her sister-in-law that they would have to leave for a while because the doctors were coming to see Mr. Lenz. "So I left," Mrs. Lenz said. She had walked down the corridor outside the ICU. In a few minutes her sister-in-law joined her. By the time they reached the end of the corridor a Code 7 had sounded. The number seven was flashing high on the wall. "And then we ran back," she said. They stood in the doorway, watching from a distance, "and we saw them running into Arthur's room."

When Yanko asked whether she could see the nurse who had been untangling her husband's IV tubing in the courtroom that day, Mrs. Lenz identified Leonora Perez. She couldn't remember her name, she said, but, "She's got the orange outfit on."

Her sister-in-law, Angie Mason, made the same identification. She had been bathing the incision across her brother's stomach, she said. It was draining and making him sore. At about three-thirty or four o'clock the nurse had come in to tell them they had to leave the room. Her brother hadn't wanted her to leave. It seemed to her that he was frightened. "He begged me not to go," she said. But the nurse insisted.

"When you left the room where was the nurse?," Yanko asked.

"She was in my brother's room."

She remembered starting toward the door leading to the corridor. The door didn't open automatically as it always did, and she had nearly crashed into it. Embarrassed, she turned to see whether anyone had noticed this and had seen doctors near her brother's room. Minutes later she saw the emergency light begin to flash.

* * *

Several times in cross-examining witnesses the defense attorneys had alluded to the unreliable nature of memory, suggesting that any number of factors could alter what a person recalled. Strong emotion, the passage of time, and the sameness of days spent in the hospital visiting a patient might lead to confusing one day with another, one event with another. Possibly it was the difficulty of remembering a painful time that had led Mrs. Lenz and Mrs. Mason to give testimony at odds with statements they had made earlier in interviews with the FBI and before the grand jury.

Mrs. Mason agreed that this was the case. That time had been "mortal Hell," she said. Mrs. Lenz believed that when she testified before the grand jury she had failed to mention Mrs. Perez alone in the room with her husband because "my nerves were all upset and my days were all combined into one." But now she had calmed down. She was sure the events of the fifteenth were as she had just reported them.

Pamela Wilson, the head nurse in charge of the day shift in the ICU, had a very different memory of events. On the afternoon of Mr. Lenz's arrest, she testified, nursing shifts were changing. The three-thirty to midnight shift was coming on duty, and she and Mrs. Perez, who was head nurse on the later shift, had been in the conference room discussing the patients in the unit. That was around four o'clock. Then they went on "walking rounds," making a tour of the patients they had discussed and stopping in Mr. Lenz's room to check on him. She was with Mrs. Perez until Dr. Bishop arrived to talk about transferring Mr. Lenz to another floor. Leaving Mrs. Perez and Dr. Bishop standing outside Mr. Lenz's room discussing the transfer, she returned to the monitoring station to complete her charting for the day.

"I hadn't been there long," she said, "when I heard someone announce that Mr. Lenz couldn't breathe and we should call a Code."

"So," attorney Stein said when he began his cross-examination, "you had been with Mrs. Perez from the time in the conference room until the time Dr. Bishop came in. And you left her with Dr. Bishop?"

Ms. Wilson nodded. "Yes."

In his hospital chart Arthur Lenz's arrest is recorded as having occurred at 4:40 that afternoon. Mrs. Perez was seen conferring with Dr. Bishop when the arrest began. She had been with Pamela Wilson for a half hour or more prior to this meeting. Yet Lenz's wife and sister remembered Perez untangling his IV tubing sometime between three-thirty and four o'clock. They remembered that she had been alone in his room when they left him and that a Code 7 had begun flashing in the corridor outside the ICU only minutes later.

Given the inconsistencies the defense had already demonstrated in the two women's testimony, it seems unlikely that their version of events was entirely persuasive, contradicted as it was by Pamela Wilson's testimony and weeks earlier by Dr. Bishop's. But now came testimony that appeared to lend weight to their version. Bonnie Weston was called to the witness stand.

CHAPTER 46

Bonnie Weston had been a nurses' assistant in the ICU during the summer of 1975. She was, in fact, the assistant O'Brien had mentioned in his opening statement as a possible suspect in the case, the one who was granted immunity from prosecution for reasons not explained. Now she sat primly in the witness chair, hands folded, a tall, blonde woman with a cautious demeanor.

On the fifteenth of August, late in the afternoon, she had been taking patients' vital signs, she said—their temperatures, blood pressure readings, and so on—going from one patient to another. Passing Mr. Lenz's room, "I just kind of glanced out of the corner of my eye," she said, "and saw Mrs. Perez in Mr. Lenz's room, apparently checking IVs." Only a minute later she heard that Mr. Lenz was having trouble breathing. Then she heard someone say, "Call a Code."

But this was not what she told the grand jury. When attorney Burgess began his cross-examination he pointed out that in her sworn testimony she said she had seen two people in Mr. Lenz's room, Mrs. Perez and a woman resembling Pam Wilson.

"At the time I said that, there was a bit of confusion in my mind as to time," Weston replied.

Burgess appeared astounded. He turned to Judge Pratt. "Your Honor, I would like a short recess to look something up in the Grand Jury transcript . . . [as] this has, frankly, come a little bit by surprise." In fact, the defense attorneys said later, the testimony had left them "flat-footed." It was entirely different from the testimony Weston had given the grand jury, entirely at odds with the testimony they had believed would benefit their case.

Fifteen or twenty minutes later Burgess returned to the courtroom. Again he confronted Weston with the contradictions in her testimony. She remained firm. She had been confusing two separate occasions, she said. Earlier that afternoon she had seen Mrs. Perez and another nurse in Mr. Lenz's room. On the later occasion she had seen only Mrs. Perez.

When Yanko returned to begin redirect examination, he asked, "And the time when you saw Mrs. Perez alone was one, two minutes before the actual event?"

"Yes, sir."

"Are you certain of that in your mind at this time?"

"Yes, sir."

So either Mrs. Perez had been with Dr. Bishop just prior to Mr. Lenz's arrest or she had been alone in his room. To further confuse matters, an entry in Lenz's medical chart stated that at 4:30 on the fifteenth of August he was complaining of shortness of breath and chest pain. His physician, questioned by the prosecution, testified that he knew of no such complaints and had heard nothing like that from Lenz. But there was the entry in the chart.

The entry was signed "L. Perez, R.N."

CHAPTER 47

In his opening statement Yanko had promised the jurors that the events of August 15 would unfold like "a living nightmare." "Lightning will strike five times," he had told them, and, as testimony moved from Lenz's arrest to Jordan Olson's almost simultaneous emergency, lightning strikes seemed an apt description.

On the fifteenth, while Lenz's resuscitation was in progress, a patient's call light began flashing above the door to the CCU. A nurse who had been standing outside Lenz's isolation room that afternoon testified that Miss Narciso had left Lenz's emergency to go to the patient in the CCU. When she returned she said that the patient, Mr. Olson, seemed apprehensive. She thought he needed extension tubing connected to his IV line to make him more comfortable and able to move more freely.

Olson's apprehension was mentioned again when Dr. Goodenday began her testimony. Olson had appeared anxious, she said, and because she was concerned about him, she had gone to the CCU to check. There was a nurse standing beside his bed but not a nurse she could identify. The woman had dark hair. She was small-boned and slightly plump and could have been Asian. But Goodenday had not seen her clearly because light coming through a window was in her eyes.

Goodenday had bent down to speak to Olson. Then she had seen he was having trouble breathing and asked the nurse to go for an airway and an ambu bag. "[A]nd she appeared frozen, she didn't move," Goodenday said. She herself had called into the corridor for help.

Bonnie Weston had seen the flashing light outside the CCU as well. When she was called again to testify, she described entering the unit and seeing Narciso beside the patient's bed. Narciso had then left the room and returned with extension tubing, which she attached to Olson's IV line. But this was before Olson was in trouble, Weston said, before his arrest.

Weston had no recollection of Dr. Goodenday being in the unit when Mr. Olson's emergency began. She remembered Dr. Hill being there and a man in a green scrub suit leaving the room just prior to the emergency, but she had not seen Dr. Goodenday.

As the contradictions began to be pile up, Yanko unexpectedly moved to a new subject. "Mrs. Weston," he said, "were you granted immunity from prosecution in this case?"

Weston nodded. "Yes, sir, I was."

"And what do you understand that to mean?"

"[T]hat if there were any definite conflicts between my testimony the first and second time at the Grand Jury, that I could not be prosecuted for perjury." This was on the advice of her lawyer, she said.

During further questioning by Yanko it became evident that the grant of immunity extended far beyond what Weston had originally stated. "It was my understanding," she said, "that I would not be prosecuted if I were involved in the murders."

She knew she was a suspect, she said. During cross-examination she spoke of the intense pressure the FBI agents had exerted, telling her at one point, "If you didn't do it, you know who did." "But that's impossible," Weston said, "because I didn't know who did it and I did not do it myself."

She had met with Dr. Lindenauer, the chief of staff, prior to her appearance before the grand jury. "He asked me to search my heart and mind for certain facts," she said. He seemed to imply that he could provide her with a promotion she coveted if she was helpful with her memories. She had regarded this as an attempt at bribery.

On her wedding day the agents had told her husband-to-be that he was marrying a liar. She had been accused of unprofessional behavior in her care of patients. She had been alone in the CCU with Mr. Olson not long before he arrested. In all she felt she would have been the defendant in the case "if things hadn't worked out just a little bit differently." But she strenuously denied that immunity had been granted to ensure that the testimony she gave would be favorable to the prosecution.

At the end of what had been a long and grueling cross-examination, Judge Pratt ordered a recess. The jurors left the room, but Weston remained on the witness stand. She had begun to cry.

After a moment Narciso rose from the defense table and went to Weston's side. Speaking softly, she poured the sobbing woman a glass of water and offered her a mint. Agent Russo rose and hurried to interrupt the colloquy. Weston, still sobbing, was led from the courtroom.

Attorney Delonis strongly objected to this behavior. A defendant was not to approach a witness, he said. Narciso had reduced the witness to tears. He called it intimidation, although Weston denied that Narciso had said anything to cause her to cry. O'Brien apologized to the court and promised that nothing of the sort would happen again. Then, at Yanko's request, Dr. Goodenday was recalled to the stand to declare that Bonnie Weston was not the nurse she had seen at Olson's bedside on the afternoon of his arrest.

* * *

"8:00 a.m. driving to Detroit. Yesterday Bonnie Bates Weston was on the stand as well as Lucy Goodenday. The defense tore into Bonnie. They brought up that the Chief of Staff had attempted to bribe her with a promotion prior to her grand jury testimony and Bonnie discussed this on the witness stand despite the prosecutors' objections. The cross-examination was by O'Brien who evidently finally got his chance to take a swipe at the Chief of Staff. All this could have been prevented if Yanko had prepared Bonnie for this possibility, but unfortunately Yanko had not."

CHAPTER 48

Later that day chemists from the FDA testified that the results of the tests they had conducted led them to believe beyond any reasonable doubt that Pavulon was present in Jordan Olson's urine sample. They had found the substance in Robert Lippy's urine as well.

Lippy, the third patient to arrest in the ICU on August 15, was being treated for a severe infection related to a self-inflicted gunshot wound, a suicide attempt that had done significant damage to his liver and kidney. While the doctors were still gathered at Olson's bedside, Lippy had begun to have difficulty breathing. Later he claimed he had seen a dark-haired man in a green scrub suit leaving his room as the arrest began.

Verna Lippy had been with her son all that day, she told Yanko, clasping her hands and leaning forward in the witness chair. She was a small, thin woman wearing a denim skirt and a rumpled cotton blouse. Her voice was tremulous. Toward five o'clock she had needed to leave the room to make a phone call, she said. "And my son says, 'Mom, don't leave me.' He kept saying, 'Don't leave me.'" Her voice shook with emotion.

But as Lippy was pleading with her not to go, Perez and Narciso walked into the room. "[A]nd that's when I felt I could leave," Mrs. Lippy said. "I felt he was being taken care of and I could go make my phone call."

Mrs. Lippy recognized these nurses as her son's regular caregivers, she said. Perez, whom she called "the little one," was going to give her son a shot. P.I. was going to attend to his IV bag.

As they had with other witnesses, the defense attorneys, on cross-examination, compared the testimony Mrs. Lippy had just given with statements she had made during her FBI interviews and grand jury testimony.

In that testimony, Stein reminded her, she had said that before she left her son's room she had seen the nurse give him a shot in his arm. In the statement given to the FBI only seven days after her son's arrest she had said that the nurse left the room before she did and when she herself departed she passed a man in the doorway, just entering. He was wearing a green scrub suit.

None of this had been included in her testimony in court that day, and Stein seemed to be suggesting that a recent meeting she had with a government attorney may have served to alter her memory of events. Certainly her failure to say on this day that she had, in fact, seen the needle enter her son's arm would serve the prosecution's argument for a bolus injection into the IV tubing. Also her failure to mention the man in the scrub suit whom she had seen entering the room as she left would remove a possible suspect from the event.

Mrs. Lippy appeared rattled as Stein continued. "[Y]ou noticed that your son was unable to talk," he said.

"Couldn't breathe."

"And he was trying to show you with his left hand what had happened?"

"His thumbs. That was it."

"And you stated [to the FBI] seven days after it happened that he made a movement with his hands as if he were using a plunger or a syringe."

"Yes."

"And you stated . . ."

Yanko rose. "Objection. At this point, Your Honor, I want to approach the bench before we go any farther."

The government's objection was related to the FBI statement Stein intended to read aloud. It contained Mrs. Lippy's description of a "conversation" she had had with her son after she returned to his room. She had asked him several questions, and he had responded by moving his head. The government attorneys were claiming that this was hearsay and inadmissible. The defense attorneys, of course, disagreed. Robert Lippy's nods, they argued, could be considered admissible.

On Monday morning Judge Pratt overruled the prosecution's objection. Stein could continue to pursue his inquiry based on Mrs. Lippy's statement to the FBI.

Accordingly, referring to the statement, Stein went on, "After you came into your son's room and he made plunger or syringe motions with his thumbs, you asked him 'Did somebody give you a shot?'"

"And he couldn't respond," Mrs. Lippy said.

But apparently he *had* responded. In her statement to the FBI she had said that her son nodded yes, Stein reminded her.

"He tried," Mrs. Lippy said, "He couldn't hardly move."

Then she asked him if it had been a nurse who gave him the shot, Stein said, and Lippy had shaken his head no.

"Oh, he couldn't. He couldn't." Mrs. Lippy was wide-eyed and trembling as Stein continued. "You asked him, 'a doctor?' And your son nodded 'no' —And then, Mrs. Lippy, you asked your son, 'Was it somebody you don't know?' And he nodded 'yes' didn't he Mrs. Lippy?"

"He tried," she whimpered. "He tried."

CHAPTER 49

The afternoon of the fifteenth had been quiet on 5West. Late that afternoon Earline Fuller, the nurses' assistant on the ward, made rounds with Phyllis Feenstra, the nurse in charge. They found their patients resting comfortably. There seemed to be no problems.

Fuller sat in the witness chair looking straight at Yanko. She was a dark-skinned woman with a forthright manner. She spoke clearly, saying she recalled that sometime between five and five-thirty she had been standing at the nurses' station in the hall on 5West when she saw Filipina Narciso approaching along the corridor from 5East. Fuller guessed she was coming from the utility room located there or from the stairwell. They waved.

"And did you believe, at that moment, that she was coming to see you?," Yanko asked.

"Well, I didn't know if she was coming to see me."

But Narciso approached, and they had a brief conversation. Narciso needed an IV solution, she said. Fuller told her to look in the 5West utility room. Narciso walked off, starting down a short hall that branched off the main corridor.

"Why did she go there?," Yanko asked. It was evident from a chart displaying the layout of 5West that this was not the way to the 5West utility room but rather led to patients' rooms, which opened onto the hall.

Fuller didn't know why, but she said that when Narciso was some ways down the short hall she called out, "Hey, Earline, what's with this patient?" She meant Sheldon Rose, Fuller said, a patient in one of the four-bed rooms.

"I said, 'Oh, he just had a suppository.'" Rose had had a fever that afternoon and had been given a suppository containing Tylenol or aspirin intended to bring down his temperature, she said. As the medication took effect and the fever broke, he had begun to perspire heavily, and Fuller thought this was what Narciso was noticing.

"She said, "Well, I don't think he looks good. I think you better come and check him.'"

"So what did you do?"

"I went down and checked." And then she reported to Feenstra that P.I. thought Rose didn't look good. Feenstra told her to take his vital signs, and Fuller returned to his room to check his pulse and blood pressure.

"Then what did you observe?," Yanko asked.

"I noticed he was having problems, you know, breathing."

Fuller had been interviewed by the FBI when the investigation began, she said, and she had told the agents about the events on 5West that afternoon, about Narciso's visit and Rose's arrest and the death that was discovered on the floor a short time later. She had told Narciso about the interview.

"How did Miss Narciso react?

"Well, she was upset . . . [and] she said, 'No Earline, that's not the way it happened. Would you tell them?' And I said, 'Well, this is the way I remember it—and this is what I told them and this is what I have to say.'"

Yanko paused. "You say she was upset?"

"Well, she was in tears—almost."

Had she told the FBI that Miss Narciso alerted her to Mr. Rose's problem while she herself was standing at the nurses' station?

Fuller said she had.

"[A]nd what did she say?"

"She said, 'No, that wasn't the way it happened.' She said, 'Remember you were down taking vital signs when I came down and spoke to you.'"

"So she stated you were down there first—and she came down to meet you?"

"Yes. But I told her 'no,' that I couldn't change my statement because—I remembered it the way I told them and that was it."

Fuller said she hadn't felt she was being pressured. She didn't feel P.I. was pleading. The conversation was simply as she now reported it.

Had she seen Miss Narciso go into Mr. Rose's room?, O'Brien asked on cross-examination. She had not. Had she watched Miss Narciso's progress down the hall every minute? She thought she had. "Do you know of any medical way that you can give a patient an injection while you're standing out in the hallway looking in on them?," O'Brien asked.

"No." Fuller almost smiled, but her smile faded when O'Brien reminded her of the report that she had been the African American nurses' assistant seen in Douglas Berry's room just prior to his Code being called.

"It's no fun to have a finger pointed at you when you didn't do something," O'Brien said. "Isn't that correct?"

Fuller agreed that it was. Further she agreed that Narciso had never asked her to lie to the FBI. "She thinks she is right and I think I am right," Fuller said. There were no further questions.

★ ★ ★

At ten minutes to six on the fifteenth of August, Dr. Bishop, returning to his office on 5 West and troubled by what he had witnessed in the ICU that afternoon, had stopped to check his patients on the floor. He found Joseph Dyllan dead in his bed.

Like many patients in the hospital that summer, Dyllan had had significant medical problems, Dr. Bishop testified, but he had not thought these problems were sufficient to result in sudden death that day. The nurse who had been in charge of 5 West that afternoon said much the same thing. Sometime after five o'clock she had changed the linen on Dyllan's bed and propped him up so he would be more comfortable. She left his room at about five-twenty.

"When you left Mr. Dyllan, did he appear to be near death?," Yanko asked her.

"He did not." Nor did he seem to be having any difficulty breathing.

Yet sometime between five-twenty and ten minutes to six Joseph Dyllan died. And Earline Fuller had seen Filipina Narciso wandering the halls on the fifth floor between five and five-thirty.

CHAPTER 50

On the twenty-sixth of May, Dr. Lee Weatherbee, the chief of laboratory services at the VA, took the witness stand to testify that blood and bile samples had been collected during Joseph Dyllan's autopsy. These had been sent to a toxicology laboratory in Denver to be tested for Pavulon because the laboratory at the VA was not equipped to perform such tests. "And they [the test results] were negative, were they not?," Stein asked.

They were negative for Pavulon, Weatherbee said, a finding that conflicted with the results of tests reported by FBI chemist Roger Aaron. Aaron had found "a foreign substance consistent in every way with Pavulon in the tissues salvaged from Dyllan's liver and lung following exhumation.

As he had earlier testified, Aaron had spent five months devising a procedure for detecting pancuronium in embalmed tissue specimens. The prosecutors were quick to point out that the Colorado laboratory had apparently spent no more than an hour and a half analyzing Dyllan's blood and bile, and the forensic chemist who had performed the analysis testified that Aaron's tests were "100 to 1,000 times better than mine." His was a simple, one-step procedure, he said. More elaborate testing could have cost the hospital as much as $250,000, whereas the simple test had cost $90.

On cross-examination Stein asked, "Are you saying that the VA hospital, with all that was going on at that time, asked you to perform a cheap test?"

The chemist would not characterize the situation that way, but there were always financial restrictions, he said. He could have run more complicated tests, but he was not asked to do so.

Overall, testimony concerning the Denver analysis did little to bolster the case for the defense. Aaron's test results were clearly more persuasive. The attorneys fared better with testimony regarding Sheldon Rose's arrest.

Rose's physician reluctantly agreed that the arrest could have resulted from a heart attack. Roger Aaron testified that he was unable to say with any certainty that he had detected pancuronium in Rose's blood plasma. And Dr. Anne Hill, called again to testify, said that when she tested Rose with the peripheral nerve stimulator she "was able to say that there was no sign of a non-depolarizing block [such as Pavulon] present in Mr. Rose at that time." She could not say whether or not the drug had been there earlier.

That morning Hill had given a riveting account of the earlier events in the ICU on August 15. As she described her decision to test the arresting patients for a paralyzing drug, the spectators in the courtroom leaned forward, obviously fascinated. They had heard much testimony implicating Pavulon in the arrests, but when this small, red-haired woman began to recount the story of her early suspicions, the testing, and the results she had obtained by administering an antidote, her testimony became as gripping as the best detective fiction.

The defense attorneys did not attempt to challenge the validity of the tests she had done. They did not challenge her statement that nothing but a nondepolarizing block could have produced the reactions the patients displayed.

Lindenauer recorded that Hill charmed everyone in the courtroom: *"Even Stein appeared mesmerized as Delonis led Anne gently through her accounts of the nerve stimulator tests and their reversals and her opinion that this had been a bolus injection given Olson. Stein very cleverly sensed the mood [in the room] and that there was really no disputing her iron-clad testimony and said up front and straightforwardly that it was clear Lippy, Olson and Lenz received a muscle relaxant!"*

Hill's conclusions were further validated when Dr. John Weg took the stand. Dr. Weg was chief of pulmonary medicine at the University of Michigan Medical Center and an expert in lung disorders. The arrests occurring at the VA in 1975 were unbelievable he said. One alone would be very, very rare, but the number of incidents that had occurred in the summer of 1975 were unexplainable, unprecedented. He, too, had concluded that the breathing failures were the result of a drug.

As testimony continued, the evidence that crimes had been committed grew steadily stronger. Dr. Michael Baden, a deputy chief medical examiner for New York City and a specialist in the causes of unnatural deaths, testified that his review of patient records led him to conclude that three patients—Howard Jackson, Joseph Dyllan, and Douglas Berry—had been murdered with a muscle-relaxing drug. Francis Foldes, an internationally known physician and expert on the effects of Pavulon, gave testimony that strongly supported the prosecution's argument for bolus injections.

Attorney Yanko, speaking later to reporters, was quoted as saying, "I don't think the jury is going to have any doubt whatsoever that crimes were committed." But he acknowledged that the evidence incriminating Perez and Narciso was not as clear-cut. "These two women are guilty," he said. "Whether they'll be found guilty or not is another question."

Stein reacted with anger, calling Yanko's comment unprofessional and saying that it was "absolutely awful" for an assistant US attorney to make such a comment. Yanko's comment appeared in headlines in the *Detroit Free Press* the next day.

CHAPTER 51

On Wednesday, June 1, after nine weeks of testimony, the attorneys for the prosecution concluded the government's case against the nurses. Shortly after noon attorney Delonis told Judge Pratt, "We now rest."

Attorneys for the defense were expected to file a motion to dismiss all charges, contending that the prosecution's evidence was insufficient to establish guilt beyond a reasonable doubt. Such motions are frequently made in criminal trials after the prosecution has finished presenting its case, but usually they are unsuccessful.

Late on Friday the defense attorneys presented the motion to Judge Pratt. In it they argued, "The total of the Government's evidence amounts to the fact that one or the other of the defendants was seen in the vicinity of some of these patients within some minutes of their medical difficulties." Under the law, mere presence was not sufficient to prove guilt, the motion stated. There was no evidence that either woman had injected a patient with a paralyzing drug, and there was no testimony that Pavulon was in the possession of either at any time. "Under these circumstances, no reasonable person could find either defendant guilty of any of the charges."

Judge Pratt scheduled a hearing for the following Tuesday. Both groups of attorneys would present arguments on the motion at that time, he said, following which he would make a ruling for or against acquittal.

On Tuesday morning, in the absence of the jury, Michael Moran began the argument for the defense, repeating much that was contained in the motion. "The defendants' presence in the vicinity of the patients is simply insufficient evidence for any juror to find guilt of conspiracy or other crimes," he said. "In order to reach that conclusion the jury would have to speculate. It would have to draw inferences from inferences."

The prosecutors countered that they had provided adequate evidence to support a guilty verdict. The instances of the nurses being repeatedly in the vicinity of the breathing failures "when taken together rise above the status of inexplicable coincidence," attorney Delonis argued.

The attorneys went through the indictment count by count, the defense asserting that in each case the evidence was inadequate, the prosecution claiming, again, that the presence of the nurses at every arrest went beyond coincidence.

Judge Pratt would need to decide whether the evidence was such that a reasonable mind might conclude guilt beyond a reasonable doubt. As he put it, "If he [the judge] concludes upon the evidence that there must be such doubt in a reasonable mind, he must grant the motion."

The original indictment charged both women with all the crimes, alleging that they were acting in a conspiracy and thus if one were guilty the other was guilty also. The next morning Pratt rejected this argument. The women were to be charged individually. Where there was no proof of active participation at a breathing failure, acquittal was granted. Thus, Leonora Perez was acquitted of the alleged poisonings of Martin, Olson, and Rose and of the murder of Jackson. No testimony had placed her at or near any of these events. Filipina Narciso was acquitted of charges that she had poisoned Mercer and Lenz for the same reason. Both nurses were acquitted on charges of poisoning Leonard Meadows and Jeffrey Wallace because Pratt felt there was insufficient evidence implicating them in either of these events, and both were acquitted of the charge that they had murdered Joseph Dyllan. "No count presents a purer case of speculation and conjecture than Dyllan," Judge Pratt said. There had been no testimony that either defendant had ever been near Dyllan's room.

Yet charges remained. Narciso was still charged with poisoning Lippy, Olson, Rose, and Martin and with the murder of Howard Jackson. Perez was charged with the poisonings of Mercer, Lenz, and Lippy. And "The conspiracy charge must stand and be presented to the jury," Pratt ruled.

Although half the charges in the prosecutors' case had been dismissed, Yanko admitted to no disappointment. "We feel the case is intact," he said. The defense attorneys also expressed optimism. "I think we all feel the best thing we have going for us in the case is Filipina Narciso and

Leonora Perez," O'Brien said. "Once the jury has a chance to see them and hear them, there certainly won't be any question in their minds."

* * *

On Thursday, the ninth of June, Judge Pratt's courtroom was filled to capacity. There was a stir of anticipation as the jurors entered. On this morning the defense would begin to call its witnesses, and the defendants themselves were expected to be the first to testify.

When the jurors were seated Judge Pratt addressed them, announcing the withdrawal of the several charges against the defendants. "You must entirely disregard all evidence which has been presented regarding these counts," he said. "Let me stress that you should not consider these withdrawals as any indication that the Court has expressed any opinion whatsoever regarding the validity of the remaining counts." Then he turned to the defense attorneys. "Who is to begin now Mr. O'Brien?"

O'Brien stood. "The defense calls Filipina Narciso."

CHAPTER 52

Narciso appeared calm as she rose from the defense table and walked the short distance to the witness stand. Smiling slightly, she settled herself and turned to O'Brien. Her evident composure and tentative smile, and even the soft gray-blue outfit she was wearing, seemed to justify O'Brien's confidence in the impression she would make. It was hard to believe that this small woman could be guilty of murder.

From the beginning the prosecutors had been faced with this skepticism. The newspapers were nearly unanimous in doubting the possibility of the women's guilt. Public opinion strongly favored their innocence. The courtroom was filled with their supporters. Yet many lawyers would agree that putting a defendant on the stand to testify in her own defense is risky. Too much can go wrong.

During cross-examination prosecutors can draw attention to the inconsistencies and apparent half truths in a defendant's testimony, comparing it to the testimony of other credible witnesses and earlier statements the defendant had made. In many instances a defendant is found guilty on the basis of his or her own testimony. But apparently the defense attorneys did not see this as a problem with regard to Filipina Narciso.

Her voice was quiet and steady as she began to speak, tinged with the accents of her native Tagalog. She gave her full name and spelled it. But people knew her as P.I., she said, because she came from the Philippine islands.

In response to O'Brien's questions she described her education in the Philippines. Since elementary school she had had an interest in nursing, she said, because her older sister, Corazon, had become an RN while she herself was just graduating from the sixth grade. She had wanted to follow in her sister's footsteps, and eventually Corazon had paid Filipina's way through nursing school.

Narciso glanced toward the back of the courtroom and smiled. Corazon was sitting with their parents in the first row of the spectators' section.

After O'Brien had established Narciso's history of employment at the Ann Arbor VA, he began a series of questions related to the individual charges she faced, starting with the poisoning charge involving Sheldon Rose. "Did you go to the fifth floor in the afternoon hours of August 15, 1975?," he asked.

"Yes," she replied. She had gone there to borrow an IV solution that was needed and not available in the ICU. She had worked on the fifth floor before transferring to the ICU and thought she would find the solution there. It was a quite common practice to borrow needed medications from other floors, she said.

O'Brien asked about her arrival on 5West. She remembered that she had seen Miss Feenstra, the RN in charge of 5West, standing near the nurses' station. She had asked to borrow the IV solution, and Miss Feenstra had told her to help herself.

"And then?"

Then she had gone to the utility room to find the solution. When she emerged, she saw Earline Fuller, the nurses' assistant on 5West, standing near the end of the short private hall that led off the main corridor. Fuller was in the process of taking temperatures, she thought. She had come out of a room with a thermometer in her hand. Already the testimony significantly disagreed with Fuller's.

They spoke, Narciso said. And then they both noticed that a patient in one of the rooms was perspiring heavily. This was because he had been given a suppository, Ms. Fuller told her.

"Did you suggest to her that she might have someone check the patient?"

"I believe I did say that."

"What did Earline Fuller do?"

"She started toward the nurses' station. I believe we walked together."

"When you got there what did you do?"

"I went down to the ICU."

A short time later she learned that Sheldon Rose had stopped breathing.

Narciso agreed that her memory of events differed from Fuller's. After the investigation began, they had had a conversation about what Fuller told the FBI. "I was kind of surprised," Narciso said. "I said, 'Well, Earline, that's not what happened—and she indicated to me some doubt like saying, 'I don't know, it might have been some other day.' So I said, 'Well, Earline, if you're not sure would you please straighten this out with the FBI?' We talked over and over again, what she remembered and what I remembered."

But she had not been angry with Fuller, she said. She had not been threatening, and she had never intended that Fuller should lie to the FBI.

O'Brien did not pursue this further. He moved on to the charge that she had poisoned Bart Martin. Here, again, her testimony differed from others' concerning Martin.

She remembered going to collect his dinner tray. He was sitting up in bed, eating slowly because he was having trouble swallowing. But she had no memory of asking the nurses' assistant in the ICU to watch him while she went to get something to eat.

"Was Mr. Martin on an IV at that time?," O'Brien asked.

"I don't recall seeing an IV."

In reviewing his chart, had she not seen a note that his IV had been discontinued?

She had. She had seen a "DC" in the chart, indicating "discontinued."

And, O'Brien asked, if a patient did not have an IV running, how would a nurse give him an injection of medication? Obviously it would not be in the way the prosecution was claiming.

It would be in the arm or the hip, Narciso said. She would have to clean the area to be injected with rubbing alcohol. She would have to explain to the patient what she was going to do.

"If you go up to Mr. Martin without telling him and just give him an injection, what do you think the most likely response would be?"

Narciso smiled broadly. "He'd probably hit me."

The spectators chuckled, but their laughter faded quickly as O'Brien moved on to the murder charge.

CHAPTER 53

Howard Jackson had died on the evening of July 30 in a room on 5West. Narciso remembered that she and Leonora Perez had left the ICU that evening to visit patients on the fourth and fifth floors, patients they had cared for. They stopped on the fifth floor to visit Mr. Haber, but seeing that the patient was not doing well and Mrs. Haber was clearly concerned, they had not stayed long.

They had gone next to 4West to visit Chester Rice. When they arrived there a nurses' assistant on the floor told them that Mr. Rice was having a serious problem. It appeared that a cut-down tray would be needed by the doctors attending to the emergency, and Narciso ran to the ICU to obtain one. She had not thought to look for one on 4West, she said. Not all floors had that kind of equipment, and as an ICU nurse she was responsible for supplying what was needed. So she ran.

"Did you ever return to the fifth floor west wing that evening?," O'Brien asked her.

"No." She had not returned to the fifth floor at all, either before or after going to the ICU.

"Did you in fact go into any other patient's room on that floor that night."

"No, I did not."

She had not gone into Mr. Jackson's room. She had not been present at his Code. Although Mrs. Haber had earlier testified that she had seen Narciso alone on 5West shortly before the Jackson Code was called, and had seen her wave as she passed by in the corridor, Narciso did not remember it that way. She had been on 5West with Leonie Perez. They had stopped to speak with Mrs. Haber some time before the Jackson Code was called. She had not been there alone.

O'Brien moved on. "Now we go ahead into August, and up to the fourteenth of August," he said. "Do you remember working that day?"

Narciso remembered that she had been working and that a Code had been called sometime after 10:00 p.m. She had left the ICU to respond, but when she reached the floor where the emergency was occurring she had not seen a crash cart in the hall or many people in the corridor. She hadn't known where to go. Then she saw a nurses' assistant rush into a darkened room. She followed her, and, although she found no Code procedure in progress, the patient in the room was clearly in trouble. The assistant began mouth-to-mouth resuscitation. Narciso started cardiac massage. Soon other people began rushing into the room.

Did she know why the nurses' assistant had gone into the room in the first place?, O'Brien asked.

"I heard later that she heard a scream from another nursing assistant," Narciso said.

Once again her memory conflicted with earlier testimony. According to that testimony, it was Narciso who had apparently discovered Douglas Berry in distress and had been the one to call for help.

Moving on to Jordan Olson's arrest, Narciso said she had added extension tubing to his IV line to make him more comfortable. This was shortly before his arrest. "But did you inject him with any medication?," O'Brien asked. "Did you inject his IV line with any medication?" Narciso answered no to both questions.

Similarly she denied injecting Robert Lippy with any medication and said she had not been in his room in the five to ten minutes preceding his arrest, although Lippy's mother had testified to seeing both Narciso and Perez in the room not long before the arrest began.

Next O'Brien pointed out that, although the defendant had known once the investigation began that she was suspect, she had made no attempt to leave the city or the country as a guilty person might have done. She had endured pressure to confess from both the FBI and the hospital administration but had refused to confess to what she had not done.

More than once O'Brien had referred to the relentless pressure brought to bear on Narciso by the government agents, the long hours of interrogation, and tactics he characterized as shocking, revolting, and a blatant violation of her rights. Now, as he began to bring his questioning to a close, he asked, "Did you inject any of the patients named in the indictment with Pavulon or any other muscle relaxant?"

"No, I did not."

"Is your conscience clear?"

"Yes, it is."

"Are you innocent of these charges?"

"Yes." Narciso nodded vigorously.

O'Brien had no further questions.

CHAPTER 54

"You were with Bart Martin prior to his arrest?," Yanko asked, looking at Narciso as he leaned forward on the podium.

The cross-examination was in its second day. Yanko had spent the first day addressing the working conditions that nurses at the Ann Arbor VA had endured in the summer of 1975. Dwelling on problems of understaffing, he had led Narciso to agree that this was a problem for both the nursing staff and the patients. In other hospitals, she said, the ratio was usually one nurse to one or two patients.

"And, instead, in the Intensive Care Unit didn't you in fact have one nurse for every four, five or six patients?"

"Most of the time."

"And in addition to that, at the time that all these Codes were going on—this magnified the situation? Caused longer hours?"

"Sometimes."

"[W]as it your feeling as a nurse that the Administration should have responded to that situation by adding people?"

Narciso felt it should have. The nurses in the ICU were bothered by the increase in Codes, she said. They questioned the cause. They wondered what was going on. Although they had talked to their supervisor, they never got an answer. But these problems had not caused her to dislike working at the VA. She had enjoyed working there until she was transferred out of patient care and assigned to a clerical job. "Otherwise," she said, "I would have quit a long time ago."

Newspapers, reporting on this first day of cross-examination, proposed that Yanko's narrow focus on overwork and understaffing represented the prosecution's attempt to establish a motive for the attacks on patients. Although the prosecutors had never publicly discussed the question of motive, sources had earlier predicted that the government attorneys would seek to suggest that the attacks were a protest aimed at the hospital administration and its failure to address the nurses' concerns.

Yanko returned to this subject when he began questioning Narciso the following morning. Then he took up the circumstances of Bart Martin's arrest.

When she was with Martin prior to his arrest had he been awake, alert, and stable?, Yanko asked.

Narciso nodded. "Yes."

"You didn't have any feeling that he was going to stop breathing?"

"No."

"You were surprised by this arrest?"

She had been, she said.

"But you requested Lula Balls to watch over him?"

"I don't recall that. Could have been."

"All right. If she's correct that you asked her, then you would have seen Martin before and determined that she should watch him?" Yanko seemed to be implying that the question was why she would have asked Balls to do this if Martin appeared to be in good shape.

"You did indicate that you remembered being with him when you went to pick up his tray? And that was a short time before his arrest?"

"Yes, in the neighborhood of five to ten minutes."

"Where was his IV line?"

She didn't remember seeing an IV line. She had seen a note in Martin's chart marked DC, or "discontinued."

Yanko asked whether she had seen a doctor's order to discontinue in the chart.

She had not.

"What would you think of a good nurse discontinuing an IV without a doctor's order?"

It was common practice to discontinue if the IV line had become detached somehow, had fallen out of the vein or been pulled out by the patient, she said. A nurse could restart the IV after contacting the doctor, but she had never seen a nurse start an IV without a doctor's order.

Even if a patient such as Mr. Martin had a "keep open" line ordered for him in case an emergency occurred?, Yanko asked.

"If that happened then the nurse can restart it, because it has been started [originally] by the doctor."

"Didn't you say two minutes ago that you had never seen a nurse start an IV without a doctor's order?"

Narciso began to seem agitated. "Did I not just tell you that . . ."

Yanko interrupted. "Didn't you say that?"

"Yes."

Mrs. Balls had testified to seeing Miss Narciso at Martin's bedside. "Did you have Pavulon with you at the time?"

"No."

"Where would you have kept it if you did have it?"

"I didn't have it."

Could she have carried a syringe concealed in the pocket of her uniform? Yanko asked. A small syringe, one that could contain the two milligrams of Pavulon needed to cause an arrest? "If you had that type of syringe in a pocket, nobody would be able to notice, would they?"

Then he asked whether a medication could be injected into an IV line and remain there, not entering the patient's bloodstream, until the flow control clamp was opened. "How long does it take to move that clamp and start the IV running?"

"Seconds."

"Five seconds? Ten seconds? You were with Mr. Martin for that period of time weren't you?"

Yes, she had been.

And she had intended to leave the CCU that evening in order to have dinner with Mrs. Perez?

She had left the unit to go to the ICU.

Evidently she didn't remember saying that she wanted to leave to get something to eat, just as she didn't remember asking Lula Balls to watch Martin, Yanko said drily. Then he asked whether Martin's arrest had upset her. "Did you feel a Code should not have been called? Didn't you tell someone that they should not have called a Code for him, and that they should have left him to die?"

Yanko's question echoed in the silent courtroom. Quietly Narciso said, "No."

CHAPTER 55

Already the morning had begun to seem long though it was not much past ten-thirty when Yanko took up the next charge. "On July 30th you left the Intensive Care Unit?," he asked.

Narciso agreed that she had.

"July 30 was the first night that a patient outside of Intensive Care received an injection of Pavulon, true?"

"I don't know."

"You went to 5West to visit Mr. Haber you said? . . . And then on to 4West to visit Mr. Rice, correct?"

"Mrs. Perez and I visited those patients that night."

"[W]hen you went to visit it was quiet? —No problem [in the ICU] with patients needing constant care? No problem with the possibility of a sudden, unexpected emergency?"

Narciso seemed undisturbed by the implication that she had been neglectful of her duties when she left the ICU that night. The patients had been stable, she said.

"When you got to Rice . . ."

When she and Mrs. Perez arrived on 4West and asked to see Mr. Rice, the nurses' assistant on the floor had told them that he was having a problem.

"And you wanted a cut-down tray, so you picked up the phone and dialed [the ICU]."

"No, I did not. I went down to the ICU and got the cut-down tray myself."

She hadn't looked for one in the utility room on 4West even though she was familiar with that floor?

She hadn't thought to look there.

"Never occurred to you?" Yanko raised his eyebrows. "When you returned from the Intensive Care Unit, did you take a detour? Did you go to 5West?"

"I did not."

"Up to this time you had been with Mrs. Perez, correct?"

They had visited Mr. Haber, had gone to 4West, and had separated when Narciso went to the ICU.

"And isn't this when Mrs. Haber saw you alone in the hallway going toward Mr. Jackson's room?"

"I did not go back to 5West."

"Didn't you wave to her?"

"That's what she testified."

"But she's wrong?"

"I did not go to 5West."

So she had returned to 4West with the cut-down tray, Yanko said. "Then the Jackson Code was called, correct? About five minutes later?"

It was a short time later, but she had not gone to that Code because she was with Mr. Rice.

"Didn't Mrs. Haber indicate that she saw you and Mrs. Perez at the end of the Jackson commotion?"

"That's what she testified?"

"[B]ut what she said was wrong again?"

"I believe Leonie and I went to see Mr. Haber before Mr. Rice's Code was called."

The press, reporting on that day's cross-examination, characterized Yanko's approach as intimidating, a mixture of accusations and questions delivered in strident tones. Whether or not this was an accurate description, he seemed unable to shake Narciso's composure. When he moved on to the fourteenth of August and Douglas Berry's arrest, she continued to answer his questions calmly.

Yanko pointed out to her that her testimony to the grand jury conflicted in several instances with answers she had given in response to O'Brien's questioning. Did she remember saying that while Codes were going on she liked to check other patients in the area who might be apprehensive, and, doing that, she had walked into Mr. Berry's room and discovered him in trouble? She'd "hollered" across the hall for help was what she had told the grand jury.

If, as she had testified, she didn't know where the original Code was taking place, "Why would you holler across the hall for help?," Yanko asked.

Narciso had no answer for this.

"Who discovered Berry, Miss Narciso?"

It was the nurses' assistant that she had followed into Mr. Berry's room, Narciso said, or the nurses' assistant who had screamed out an alert just prior to that. Evidently she had no memory of telling the grand jury that she had found Berry in trouble and called for help herself. As had been the case a number of times in her replies to Yanko, she simply didn't remember.

CHAPTER 56

"Yanko had some carefully laid traps for Narciso and comments were that her demeanor changed significantly when he began cross-

examining her. O'Brien had her bouncy and relaxed and pleasant. Her answers came forward almost before a question was asked. She turned somber when Yanko started his cross-exam and was slow to unwind. Earlier O'Brien and Narciso had touched on the Chief of Staff and said that I had asked Narciso to confess. A long discussion with Yanko ensued after court was over about how to handle this. I have no idea what he is going to do.

"I should say I am excluded from the courtroom. In an in-chamber conference it was said that I should stay out of court since I might be called to testify."

Potential witnesses were not allowed in court to hear other witnesses testify. This was routine. But in Lindenauer's case the banishment seemed especially pointed. There was no certainty that he would be called as a witness for the prosecution, and in fact he never was. Nevertheless, the defense attorneys objected to his presence in the room, complaining to the judge that he had "coached" witnesses. On more than one occasion the judge had asked him to leave.

"I recall one specific instance when at a break I was leaning over the prosecutor's table, pointing out something in a record to a prosecution witness. Stein, who was always annoyed at my participation, complained of coaching. Despite vigorous denials by Delonis, the judge told me to leave the courtroom."

When Yanko continued his cross-examination that morning, he turned to the events that had occurred in the ICU on August 15, saying, "August 15 was a big day, wasn't it?"

There could be little argument with that. Already the jurors had heard abundant testimony about August 15, testimony from Arthur Lenz's wife and sister, Robert Lippy's mother, Drs. Goodenday and Hill, and a number of residents and nurses who had been present in the ICU when the Codes were called there. Further, they had heard testimony concerning events on 5West that afternoon. To call August 15 a big day seemed like a considerable understatement.

Yanko smiled as if he were aware of this. The he continued, "You went to the Lenz Code and assisted at the crash cart?"

"Yes."

"Then Olson's call light went on and you went to see him. . . . [A]nd he said he was uncomfortable, correct?"

"Yes." Narciso nodded.

"But he didn't ask for extension tubing, did he? That was *your* idea."

"That was the only thing I could do for him."

The patient had been apprehensive, she said. He could not move freely. And so she had gone to get tubing to add to his IV line so he could move more easily.

"And it was more important to you to take the time [to add the tubing] than to attend to an emergency?"

There were others, she said. The Lenz Code was well attended.

"So you put an extension tubing on Mr. Olson? You pulled the curtain around his bed?"

"I don't remember, but that is the usual thing to do if a patient is apprehensive, to give them a little privacy."

But hadn't she told the FBI agents when they questioned her that pulling the curtain might have been a mistake, causing her to look suspicious? "To your thinking is that a suspicious act?," Yanko asked.

"No." It was common practice in the unit, she said.

"But isn't it suspicious because you did it for another reason?"

"I did not do anything."

"You didn't draw the curtain or you did draw the curtain?"

"I have no memory."

"So you went back to the Lenz Code."

"I did."

"Then you returned to Olson when he began his arrest?"

"I returned when I saw Dr. Goodenday enter the room and I followed her along with other people."

"You ran to him. Correct?"

"I don't think I ran."

Yanko asked her to look at her copy of the FBI interrogation. "If you will look at page 2, the third full paragraph. It starts with 'She stated that after about five minutes [of leaving the room] Olson's light came on again and she ran to his bedside. She stated that when she arrived there Dr. Goodenday was already at the bed, but she did not see anyone else.' If you did run to Olson didn't you run because you knew what was wrong with him?," Yanko asked.

"No." Again Narciso shook her head.

In earlier testimony Dr. Goodenday had said that when she entered the CCU she had seen a nurse standing on the far side of Olson's bed. This nurse had seemed not to understand when Goodenday asked her to get an ambu bag and oxygen but had simply stood there, openmouthed.

Now Yanko asked, "Isn't it a fact, Miss Narciso, that the nurse at Mr.

Olson's bed was you? Isn't it a fact that the nurse that Dr. Goodenday spoke to and made requests of was you?"

"She did not ask me anything."

Yanko asked her to look again at the FBI report and then he read aloud, 'Narciso stated that she asked Goodenday what she could do and then Goodenday told her to get some oxygen.' "Do you recall making that statement, Miss Narciso?"

"I don't."

"And so you left, you said, to get something. I forget what."

"I went back to Lenz's Code to get a crash cart because Lenz's Code was wrapping up."

"You left Olson's room. Is that when you went to Mr. Lippy?"

"I didn't go to Mr. Lippy's room."

It was evident that Yanko had not finished his cross-examination, but it was nearing one o'clock, the usual hour to adjourn the proceedings for the day, and not much more could be accomplished in the little time remaining.

Yanko approached the bench, and after a short discussion Judge Pratt announced a recess until the following Monday morning. Admonishing the jurors, as he did each day, to refrain from discussing the trial and avoid contact with any news source, he concluded, "Enjoy your weekend. You are excused."

The jurors rose and slowly filed from the courtroom. Looking weary, Narciso rose, too, and joined the attorneys at the defense table. The room began filling with a murmur of voices as the spectators straggled toward the doors.

CHAPTER 57

On Monday morning Yanko took up where he had left off, returning to Jordan Olson's arrest. "The extension tubing you placed on Mr. Olson," he asked, "how long before his arrest did you place that tubing, Miss Narciso?"

"A short time."

"A short time, which you previously indicated was five to ten minutes."

"I would say it was under ten minutes."

But hadn't she said earlier [in an interview with FBI agent Ward] that it was twenty to thirty minutes before his arrest that she placed the tubing?, Yanko asked.

Narciso seemed confused. "It is possible."

"Why is it possible?" Yanko demanded. "If you put the extension tubing on Mr. Olson five or ten minutes before his arrest, why is it possible that you would have said that it happened twenty to thirty minutes before?"

Had she been trying to put as much time as she could between her last contact with Olson and his arrest?, he asked.

Narciso shook her head. "No," she said.

* * *

When Yanko began to address the journey Narciso had made to 5West on August 15 to obtain an IV solution needed in the ICU, there were few in the courtroom who were not familiar with it. That terrain had been covered at length by O'Brien. Although Yanko's efforts to discredit Narciso's reasons for going to 5West to obtain the solution raised questions, he elicited nothing more that would involve her in Sheldon Rose's arrest. She had been on the floor prior to the arrest, she agreed, but she had not entered Rose's room and there had been no earlier testimony to place her there.

In all, Yanko's cross-examination had spanned three days and lasted almost seven hours. As it came to a close, he said, "Miss Narciso, I have asked you frequently why someone would want to hurt these patients and I have asked you what reasons someone would have for doing this, and basically have had no explanation, correct?"

"I don't believe anyone would hurt a patient."

"Do you remember a questionnaire that was passed out in October of 1975 by doctors at the VA Hospital?"

"Yes."

"Do you recall that in response to one of the questions, you wrote that someone may have tried to do this deliberately?"

Referring her to the questionnaire, Yanko said, "Question 30 reads, 'Why do you think this person did this?' The answer, 'Someone who might be against the VA hospital.' Did you write that?"

"Yes."

Yanko nodded and stepped away from the podium. "No further questions."

* * *

On redirect O'Brien returned to the six hours the FBI agents had spent interrogating Narciso. "And have you forgotten some of the things you said then?," he asked, suggesting that the discrepancies between her testimony that day in court and the statements she had made to the FBI could be explained as simple forgetfulness.

Finally he asked, "Did you do the things you have been charged with?"

Narciso took a deep breath and turned to look steadily at the jury. "No," she said.

CHAPTER 58

At midmorning on Monday Judge Pratt called a brief recess, a needed break before the next witness was to testify. When the jurors returned, attorney Burgess called Leonora Perez to the stand.

Perez appeared calm as she took the witness chair and was sworn in. Frowning, she looked out across the courtroom. Her husband and father were sitting in the second row of the spectators' section. Her mother, as the papers reported, was at home caring for the Perez children, Christopher, four, and Jeffery, nearly seven months old now. When Burgess began his questioning, he inquired about both children before going on to ask about the years Perez had spent growing up in the Philippines.

Her family has been poor, she said. She had always had to work to help herself and them. It was much the same background that Narciso had described, but Perez seemed more assertive. She had come to the United States for a better life, she said.

Originally she had gone to Chicago to work, but eventually she and her husband had come to Michigan where she found employment at University Hospital in Ann Arbor as a permanent evening nurse. Leaving there after a time, she transferred to the VA. "Better salary, better benefits," she said matter-of-factly.

Following her orientation at the VA, she had been assigned to the afternoon shift in the ICU during the second or third week of June 1975.

Had she known Miss Narciso at the time?, Burgess asked.

"No." Miss Narciso had not been working in the ICU then. They had met only once, in a hallway during Perez's orientation.

That the two had known one another for only a short time before the arrests began was one of the defense's arguments against the conspiracy charge. As O'Brien had said in his opening statement, it seemed improbable that the two would have hatched a plot to poison patients after such a brief acquaintance. Burgess's question seemed meant to emphasize that improbability.

Besides the conspiracy charge, Perez faced three charges of poisoning. The jurors had heard testimony placing her at or near the arrests of Arthur Lenz, Robert Lippy, and Homer Mercer. Burgess began with Mercer.

"Testimony has been introduced that Mr. Mercer had a breathing problem on July 29," he said, "but a Code wasn't called for him. Were you working that night?"

"Yes, I was."

"Do you recall the incident?"

"No."

In fact she recalled nothing that agreed with the testimony Mercer's son had given. The son had never complained to her about the nursing care she had provided his father, she said. Her supervisor had never mentioned a complaint. She had not been present at his father's bedside when he arrested. She had not been at the bedside when his son shouted for help. She recalled none of that.

As for Arthur Lenz's arrest, she remembered being in the conference room at a nurses' meeting until about four o'clock on that afternoon. Following the meeting she had made walking rounds of the patients in the unit with Pam Wilson, who was going off duty. They had gone into Mr. Lenz's room together.

None of this agreed with the testimony provided by Lenz's wife and sister, who claimed that Perez had been the nurse who asked them to leave Lenz's room, the one who had been alone with him shortly before his Code was called. The testimony was, likewise, at odds with Bonnie Bates Weston's memory of having seen Perez alone in Lenz's room as she passed by.

Perez claimed that she had not told Mrs. Lenz to leave her husband's room. She had not even *been* in the room when the women were there, and she had not been alone there later. She and Miss Narciso were standing in the hall *outside* Mr. Lenz's room, talking with Dr. Bishop, when Mr. Lenz's problem began. She heard him calling for a nurse and saw him motioning toward his chest.

"What did you do?"

"I went to him."

"You went into Mr. Lenz's room alone?"

"I think P.I. went with me."

And, seeing that Mr. Lenz was having a problem breathing, she had left his room to call a doctor.

Later, on cross-examination, Delonis would ask Perez why she had to leave Lenz's room to call a doctor when Dr. Bishop was standing just outside the door.

In the case of Mr. Olson's arrest, Perez said, she had been standing at the crash cart outside Mr. Lenz's room when P.I. approached and told her that Olson was having a problem, that he was upset and apprehensive.

"And what did you do?"

"I went to check."

How soon did she go to check after Miss Narciso told her this?, Burgess asked.

"Maybe three to five minutes, something like that."

"And what did you observe when you got there?"

"He was sitting up in bed—his face was reddish. He said he was upset because of the commotion going on inside the Unit." Clearly this was not a description of a patient undergoing an arrest. Olson had been speaking and moving, and his color was far from gray-blue. At least this was what Perez claimed to remember.

She had spoken to him, she said, reassuring him, and then returned to Lenz's Code. Sometime after she returned she heard Dr. Goodenday calling for an ambu bag and oxygen and realized that Mr. Olson was in trouble, so she went to find the equipment Dr. Goodenday needed. Not long after that Mr. Lippy arrested.

"Have you been interrogated by the F.B.I. about these matters?," Burgess asked.

"Numerous times."

The agents had been mean, she said, pounding the table, demanding a confession, calling her a liar. During this time she had been relieved of her nursing duties in the ICU and transferred to the nursing office. In November 1975 she had moved back to Chicago to work at a VA hospital there.

"Why?," Burgess asked her.

"Because I could not take it any more. Too much harassment and too much interrogation."

Yet, after only one week at the hospital in Chicago, she was again relieved of her active nursing duties and assigned to the nursing office. And she was interrogated again in Chicago. "Two agents came from Detroit," she said.

"They came all the way to Chicago to interrogate you?," Burgess asked, managing to seem incredulous.

Perez nodded vehemently. "Yes."

Again they had asked her to confess. "One said, 'This will be the last time you will see your boy—your son—again.'" But she had refused to confess, she said, because she *had* nothing to confess. She was innocent.

CHAPTER 59

When Richard Delonis began the cross-examination he turned to questions about Perez and Narciso's relationship, clearly addressing the conspiracy charge. They had come to know each other while working together in the ICU?, he asked.

"Yes."

And they had much in common, Delonis suggested, both having come from the Philippines? "From time to time you even talked in your native tongue?"

"Yes, because I could speak that fluently . . ."

"So you would often talk in the Filipino language rather than in English?"

Perez shook her head. "No, We don't talk Filipino when we are in front of Americans." Some people didn't like that, she said.

"Because they wouldn't know what you were saying, I take it."

"Yes."

Delonis nodded. This appeared to be his point.

Why had she told the grand jury that she had moved to Chicago to be near relatives but had never mentioned FBI harassment?, he asked. "You did not say anything at all about F.B.I. harassment, did you?"

"No."

"Why not? Who were you afraid of?"

"The F.B.I. because of the way they treated me. I could not take it any more."

"But they weren't in the room, were they?" Delonis reminded her that her testimony before the grand jury was secret. "And you didn't mention the harassment?" Why had she not wanted to mention it?

For the first time Perez seemed uncertain. She hesitated, appearing reluctant to speak. She glanced toward the lawyers at the defense table. Then she said, "I was afraid to say it because they might fire me out of the hospital, because I know they [the FBI and the VA hospital] are from the same branch of government and I don't know the law here."

"And you cannot erase that [harassment] from your mind? But it did not occur to you to tell the grand jury about that?"

Burgess stood. "Your Honor—excuse me. He has asked the question probably ten times and ten different ways and she has responded. I think that Counsel should be instructed to go on to another line of questioning."

Judge Pratt turned to Delonis and raised his eyebrows. "Let's not become overly repetitious, Counselor."

"May I put the question just one more time, Your Honor?"

Judge Pratt agreed, and Delonis continued, "When you left Ann Arbor, Mrs. Perez, was part of your reason that you were afraid of what the F.B.I. might find out about you?"

"No. Because I never hid anything from them." Perez folded her arms across her chest, seeming to have regained her composure, determined that Delonis would not force her to say anything she did not choose to say.

* * *

The next morning Delonis began his questioning again, asking about Bart Martin and the IV line that had been detached and not replaced. Wasn't failure to keep the line attached like sending someone who couldn't swim out into the middle of a lake in a leaky boat without a life preserver?, Delonis asked.

Perez seemed confused, and Delonis, apparently annoyed, repeated the analogy. Then he said, "Let's talk for a couple of minutes about Mr. Mercer." Had she heard his son's testimony? Did she recall his description of a nurse at his father's bedside that seemed to fit her?

Perez shook her head. "It did not. I was not at the bedside."

But the description did fit her right down to the gold tooth, didn't it?, Delonis asked.

Perez sighed. "I have a gold tooth."

CHAPTER 60

"I had a number of conversations with Yanko concerning motive and pointed out that he must present a motive so that the jury will have a reason that they can look to if they wish to come in with a guilty verdict. My thoughts are that they must have a reason no matter how flimsy to allow them to justify a guilty verdict so they can live with it. I believe Yanko accepted this notion."

The prosecutors had been circling the question of motive for weeks, returning repeatedly to the problems of overwork and understaffing and to the hospital administration's failure to address the situation. Although the attorneys had not explicitly characterized the poisonings as protests meant to draw attention to working conditions in the hospital, they had frequently implied as much, leaving the jurors to infer the connection. Now, as Delonis continued his cross-examination of Perez, he left less to the jurors' imagination.

Mrs. Perez had known that Dr. Bishop was coming to the ICU on the afternoon of August 15 to negotiate Arthur Lenz's transfer out of the unit, had she not?, he asked.

Perez agreed that she had. She had spoken with Dr. Bishop on the phone about his need for a bed in the ICU.

"And of all the patients in the ICU or CCU that day, Mr. Lenz was the one in the best condition to be moved out, wasn't he?"

"I believe so."

"Okay. Now if somebody wanted to make some kind of point with the hospital administration through Dr. Bishop, let's say, by causing a respiratory arrest. Since Mr. Lenz was in the best condition, the most dramatic point would be to have him as the target, is that true?"

"Target? —I did not get your question." Perez frowned and shook her head. Sighing, Delonis explained what he meant. The nurses' seemingly incomplete command of English had repeatedly frustrated the prosecutors in their questioning.

"And sometime during Mr. Lenz's Code, Dr. Goodenday arrived, didn't she?," Delonis asked.

"I believe so."

"And shortly after Dr. Goodenday arrived, Mr. Olson had a respiratory arrest?"

In fact, by the time Jordan Olson arrested not only were Bishop and Goodenday present in the ICU, but Drs. Freier and Hill were there as well. If the poisonings were intended to make a dramatic statement to the hospital administration, the timing could not have been improved upon.

Delonis paused long enough to underline the inference. Then he addressed Jordan Olson's arrest.

Mrs. Perez had told the FBI that she had seen both Dr. Goodenday and Miss Narciso at Mr. Olson's bedside at the time of his arrest. In a later statement she had neglected to mention Miss Narciso's presence. Why was that? And, referring to Dr. Goodenday's testimony, he asked what member of the afternoon shift in the ICU on August 15 could be described as a female approximately five foot three to five foot five in height, plump, with a round face and short black hair and of Asian origin?

"I don't know," Perez replied.

"Did Miss Narciso fit that general description?"

"No."

"She did not?"

"No."

Why had Mrs. Perez told the agents she had gone to check on Mr. Olson after Miss Narciso left his room and some time before he arrested? Was she trying to protect Narciso by establishing that Narciso was not the last person with Mr. Olson? "Did you really leave the Lenz Code before the Olson Code, Mrs. Perez, or is this just a story to take Miss Narciso off the hook?"

Perez took a deep breath and looked steadily at Delonis. "I was not protecting her," she said. "I left the Lenz Code to check on Mr. Olson." When she left Olson's room the last person there was Bonnie Bates Weston, she said.

After Delonis had finished, Burgess stood quickly and turned to the bench. "If I might just have a second, Your Honor?"

Burgess seemed concerned as he stepped to the podium. Addressing Perez, he asked, did she recall a warning she had been given just prior to her first appearance before the grand jury? Hadn't she been warned that if she was withholding information or testifying falsely to protect someone else, she risked being taken from her family and put in jail? "When Mr. Delonis asked you questions regarding the description Dr. Goodenday gave us here in court, he asked whether or not the description fit Miss Narciso—. Does it fit Miss Narciso?"

"Yes."

"Okay. And why did you say it didn't?"

Perez hesitated. "Because she is my friend."

Delonis immediately returned to this conflict in Perez's testimony. "Earlier this morning when you said 'no,' you were not telling the truth, were you, to this jury?"

Perez frowned. "See, when I said 'no' it was because she's my friend and I know she's not the kind of person will do something wrong. She's a good person."

"You told the jury 'no' because you wanted to protect your friend?"

"No. I'm not protecting anybody, Mr. Delonis. She's just my friend."

"It was difficult for you to tell this jury that she fit the description, is that it?"

"It's not difficult because I said 'yes' to Mr. Burgess."

"But you didn't say that to me, did you?"

"No."

Delonis turned to the bench. "Nothing further, Your Honor."

And it seemed that nothing further was needed. Delonis had established that Perez had given false testimony to the jury. Despite her denial, it appeared obvious that the testimony was intended to protect Filipina Narciso. If it resulted in nothing more, this testimony would surely add weight to the prosecution's argument for a conspiracy.

At the end of her testimony Perez declared, as Narciso had, that she was guilty of none of the charges against her. Then she rose and returned, straight-backed and frowning, to the table where her lawyers sat.

What the jurors had made of the women's testimony was in no way apparent. Clearly they had listened attentively, but their faces remained impassive.

They had become familiar figures to the spectators in the courtroom—the bearded young fellow with his squinting eyes, the full-bosomed woman tapping her pencil thoughtfully against her cheek, the gray-haired man who sat stooping in his chair as if he bore a great weight between his shoulders. Day after day in the jury box they sat in their rumpled clothes, occasionally coughing or stifling a yawn or jotting in the notebooks Judge Pratt had provided, but whatever judgments they were making about what they had heard lay hidden behind expressionless gazes.

CHAPTER 61

O'Brien later wrote that as the trial progressed the defense attorneys discovered "a disturbing pattern" in the statements of some witnesses. "With each FBI interview," he wrote, "several witnesses seemed to alter their version of events in ways favorable to the Government." While not directly accusing the FBI agents of deliberately seeking to influence the witnesses' testimony, he does propose that witness testimony can often be shaped by postevent suggestions, especially if those suggestions come from representatives of the US government. "To counter that effect, we needed an expert who understood the dynamics of memory and eyewitness observation."

Dr. Elizabeth Loftus was such an expert. A professor of psychology at the University of Washington and the author of several books on the subject of memory and eyewitness testimony, she was called to testify by the defense. Judge Pratt required that her testimony be taken in the absence of the jury for reasons that were not immediately apparent.

Out of hearing of the jurors, Dr. Loftus spoke at length about the many sources that could contribute to an individual's memory of events. Memory did not work like a camera, she said. It could be altered and shaped in a number of ways, including by means of subtle or indirect suggestion. This was, of course, what the defense was contending. The attorneys had noted several prosecution witnesses whose accounts of events had altered following contact with government attorneys or FBI agents and could thus be considered unreliable.

But Judge Pratt was not moved to reconsider his decision to absent the jury from this testimony. Through cross-examination and argument the defense attorneys could call into question the reliability of witnesses, he said. The jurors were capable of judging for themselves without hearing the testimony of an expert witness.

When the jurors returned to the courtroom that day, the defense called the next witness.

Out of the witness room came Robert Lippy, a strapping, broad-shouldered former Marine who had served in Vietnam. Lippy was the only patient of those still surviving who claimed to remember his arrest. Although his mother had testified as a prosecution witness, Lippy had not been called.

Lippy had for several years been receiving psychiatric care at the VA in an effort to treat his depression. In the summer of 1975 he had been admitted to the hospital following a suicide attempt—a gunshot that had seriously damaged his internal organs. Now he seated himself on the witness stand and raised his right hand, preparing to testify for the defense.

Because Lippy had suffered several arrests while hospitalized, O'Brien began his questioning by establishing that the arrest about to be described had occurred on August 15 in the ICU. That done, he asked Lippy to describe the event.

He had been dozing, he said, made drowsy by the pain medication he was receiving, when suddenly he felt a pain in his arm and a tug on his IV tubing. Through hazy eyes he saw someone standing over him, a man who had his hands on the IV line. By the time his eyes focused, this person—this man in a green outfit—was on his way out the door.

Then Lippy began to panic. "I remember trying to sit up because it felt like somebody had their hands around my lungs, just squeezing out the air. I couldn't breathe," he said.

"After, I don't know how long a time it was, I managed to hit the little button that you have beside your bed if you have a problem or if you want to talk to somebody. And Pam Wilson came in."

Perez and Narciso had been in his room that afternoon, just as his mother testified, he said. Referring to them as P.I. and Leonie, he spoke of them calling a doctor to adjust his IV tubing because it had become uncomfortable. But they had left the room when his mother did, he said. They had left well before he began to have trouble breathing.

O'Brien asked whether Lippy had been interviewed by the FBI. Lippy said he had been, several times, but the agents had not appeared interested in hearing about the man in green who had been in his room. They seemed to want to talk about the nurses. "And there have been a few occasions where they have expressed that the girls are guilty and that somebody in the hospital did try to kill me—. And it frightened me. But still I don't personally believe those girls are guilty—."

O'Brien asked whether the prosecutors knew he felt that way.

Lippy nodded. "I believe so."

During cross-examination the next day, Lippy admitted to some difficulty unscrambling the events of his several arrests.

"Are you confident that what you related yesterday is how it happened?," Yanko asked.

"Correct."

But as Lippy's testimony continued, he seemed to become increasingly confused. "I had six, seven, possibly eight arrests in that hospital," he said.

So it could have been the third or fifth or seventh arrest he remembered?, Yanko asked. Despite what he had told O'Brien earlier, Lippy agreed that it could have been.

Yanko referred to statements Lippy had made to the FBI agents and to his testimony before the grand jury. "When you testified before the grand jury, didn't you indicate that P.I. and Leonie and your mother left a short time before your breathing failure, not a long time before?"

In fact it had been almost immediately before, he had told the grand jury, saying that the last person to handle his IV tubing had been P.I.

Wasn't it possible that the man in green he had mentioned had come into the room, responding to Lippy's summons for help?, Yanko asked.

"No, he wasn't summoned by me," Lippy said. "No, sir."

But he had told the grand jury that he had called for assistance, that he had pushed the call button beside his bed. "Jesus," Lippy said. "You're getting me really, really confused."

Carefully, Yanko proceeded, alluding to Lippy's suicide attempt, to his depression and his three or four years in psychotherapy. "Isn't it a fact," he asked "that your depressive state at the time of these events affected your ability to remember them?"

Lippy agreed that was possible. "But I don't like to talk about it at all," he said, and added that he had been told the FBI went into his psychiatric records without his knowledge. "That's between me and my therapist," he said angrily. "I am upset about that."

But hadn't he signed a release?, Yanko asked. "Well," Lippy replied, "if I signed something I wasn't aware of it at the time."

Yanko did not continue this line of questioning. "Isn't it a fact, Mr. Lippy, that the first time you told [any FBI agent or representative of the government] about a man standing over your bed was in your testimony yesterday?," he asked.

Lippy straightened up and frowned. "No, sir, I don't believe that is a fact."

"July 1, on my way back from Detroit: Lippy did us some damage overall. However I felt that his not being put on the witness stand was a good choice since he was so unreliable and had such a bad psychiatric history. Nevertheless the advantage that the defense gained in putting a

victim on the stand was considerable and Lippy's story could be interpreted in a variety of ways."

The prosecutors ion had not been concealing anything when they did not call Lippy to testify, they claimed. They had simply felt that his memory of events was too confused to provide useful testimony in an important case. They had discussed their reasons with him before the trial began, and he had seemed to understand. But now his mention of the lack of interest the FBI agents had shown when he spoke of the man in the green outfit seemed to indicate that the prosecutors had other reasons for deciding not to call him. O'Brien suggested as much in his questioning, giving the jurors a reason to wonder.

CHAPTER 62

Max Murphy was a small, stooped man. His wrinkled short-sleeved cotton shirt seemed too large for his small frame. He had been a patient in a room on 5West in the summer of 1975, he said. His room was just across the hall from Howard Jackson's, not more than thirty feet away, and he had often both seen and heard Jackson speaking to the doctors and nurses. Jackson was a very sick and cantankerous old man, Murphy said. He had heard him arguing and complaining and had heard him say more than once that he wanted to die.

On the evening on which Jackson *did* die, Murphy had seen a man in his room wearing one of those green scrub suits the doctors sometimes wore around the place. The man was handling Jackson's IV line. He was almost fondling it, Murphy said. "[A]nd it began to bother me a little bit. I thought, what the hell is he doing? Whatever he's doing why don't he do it and get out of there?"

Then a nurse came in. She went into Jackson's room, took the man's hand, and led him away, and Murphy could see that what he was wearing was a pair of green pajamas. Hearing what the man was saying and observing his unsteady gait, Murphy judged that he was mentally impaired.

(In fact, the man in question was a patient who had been transferred to 5West from the psychiatric floor for medical treatment. The night Jackson died, he had broken his restraints, left his room, and begun to wander.

The nurse who found him in Jackson's room had already testified about these circumstances.)

A short time later, Murphy said, another nurse entered Jackson's room, cried, "Oh my God!," and went running down the hall. Murphy could see that Jackson was slumped over.

O'Brien paused. He had a tough but important question, he said. "Do you believe, Mr. Murphy, that you observed Mr. Jackson die that night?"

"Yes."

"Would you tell us about that?"

He had seen Jackson raise up, give a loud groan, a sigh, and slump over. "I felt Mr. Jackson was gone," he said. Then he hesitated. "This is the thing I didn't want to tell. I didn't call out. I didn't say anything. He was old and sick . . . I felt let the poor old sick man die." Murphy's voice trembled with emotion as he spoke. The courtroom was silent. "If I made a bad mistake, then I made it," he said.

Earlier Murphy had said that, although there were several nurses in and out of Jackson's room that evening, he had not seen Perez or Narciso. Now O'Brien asked him to take a good look at the two women seated at the defense table. "You are sure that you did not see them on the 5th floor, west wing on July 30, 1975?"

"No, I never saw those women."

He held fast to this denial when Yanko began to question him, although he admitted that he had not been watching Jackson's room without a break that evening. Did the fact that he had not seen the defendants mean they hadn't been there?, Yanko asked.

"Oh no, sir. No." Murphy shook his head.

* * *

The defense called thirteen additional witnesses that day. They were friends, relatives, and coworkers, all of whom testified to the defendants' honesty and reliability and declared that neither would harm a patient. The youngest of these was a thirteen-year-old boy, Narciso's neighbor and her friend, he said. They went to movies together. She encouraged him to do his homework. On the day she was released on bail, he had baked a cake for her. "Can you conceive of her harming or injuring another human being?," O'Brien asked him.

The boy looked appalled. "No way. She'd never do that."

* * *

The defense had been expected to call still more witnesses, among them an expert on the effects of Pavulon who had flown from London to appear, but on Monday, June 20, surprising everyone, the attorneys announced that they rested their case.

The prosecution proceeded to call several rebuttal witnesses, most of whom had testified before. Some were called to rebut the account Perez had given concerning events in the ICU on August 15. Agents of the FBI testified, denying the claims that they had intimidated the nurses during questioning. And then there was nothing more. The jury was excused for the weekend.

On Monday, the twenty-seventh of June, Judge Pratt greeted the jurors cordially as he did each morning, then said, "We have now reached that stage in the proceedings where Counsel will present their final arguments." Cautioning that these arguments were not evidence but only the attorneys' respective theories, their interpretations of evidence, he turned and asked Yanko to begin.

But it was Delonis who began. He acknowledged that the trial had been a long one, that the witnesses had been numerous. He spoke of the prosecution's obligation to prove guilt beyond a reasonable doubt. Circumstantial evidence could on occasion be more persuasive than direct evidence, he said, and the jurors would want to bear in mind the concepts of intent and motive. The government was obliged to prove intent, establishing that the actions were done purposely, but it had no obligation to prove motive or the reasons why the action was taken.

He went on to discuss the nature of conspiracy. Conspiracy was sometimes difficult to prove, he said, but proof could be found in examining the actions of the members of an alleged conspiracy. Were they acting together? Did they appear to have a common objective?

He spoke of the individual patients listed in the indictment, enumerating the symptoms and circumstances of their arrests. Finally he asked, "Was there [in each case] a crime committed?"

He rejected the possibility of contamination in the IV bags received from the supplier. He stressed that the physicians attending the patients had seen no medical reason, nothing in the patients' condition, to produce the arrests. He spoke of Dr. Hill's nerve stimulator tests and administration of antidotes, of the FDA's discovery of Pavulon in the urine tested, of the discovery of the drug in Howard Jackson's exhumed tissues. He emphasized the excellent credentials of those who had done the testing. He recalled the testimony of expert witnesses who had dismissed the possibility of a "time bomb," or slow administration of the drug, saying that a rapid bolus injection was indicated in all events. In effect, he summarized most of the testimony the jurors had heard, saying that, indeed, poisonings had occurred, crimes had been committed.

"Now we approach the next question. Who did it? Who committed these crimes? Who was at the bedside just prior to the arrest? What were they doing? Why were they there?

"The answer to that question, ladies and gentlemen, will lead you to the identification of who was responsible and to address you as to that—I call my colleague, Mr. Yanko."

CHAPTER 63

Yanko appeared confident as he took his place at the podium. Straightening his shoulders, he looked at the jurors for a moment and then began to speak, first thanking them for their service during the long trial. "But the end is near," he said. "Soon now, very soon, you will exercise your responsibility and duty, namely to determine the innocence or guilt of the accused." He himself could count forty-three factors that suggested guilt.

There were six thousand pages of testimony, he told them. "Now, bearing in mind that it is your duty to consider all evidence, let us nevertheless review those facts which hopefully are most significant."

The jurors had heard testimony about the "tragic, appalling one month" in the hospital's history and of "the evil which lurked in the halls in search of victims. . . . If the familiarity which you have with these events has somehow diminished your awareness of the darkness of those hours, reflect for a moment on those who once lay gasping for air, struggling for their last breath."

He continued, speaking of the arrests individually. "July 29: Bart Martin. 'Enjoy your dinner, Mr. Martin!' You heard the testimony of Lula Balls, nursing assistant." Although the testimony contained uncertainties as to the timing of events, the story was simple. "Filipina Narciso was the last person to be with Martin and when she left, disaster entered. Martin had a respiratory arrest, an arrest caused by a bolus injection of

Pavulon. The injection had to have been given when Filipina Narciso was there." Miss Narciso had not challenged Mrs. Balls's version, Yanko said. She had simply declared that she didn't recall the events as Mrs. Balls had recounted them. Yanko seemed to be ignoring Narciso's claim that no IV line was in place before Martin arrested.

He pointed out that there were a great many contradictions apparent when comparing the defendants' testimony with that of other witnesses. In the case of Homer Mercer, Mercer's son claimed that Leonora Perez was the nurse at his father's bedside when he arrested. Perez denied having been there at all or having any memory of the episode. "If she was there, she is lying now, not just forgetting. For surely if she was there at that dramatic a moment, she would not forget it."

On July 30, 1975, "there were two emergencies that occurred almost back to back, within a ten to fifteen minute period of time. The first, on 4West, was for a man by the name of Chester Rice. That was followed by a second on 5West for the murdered Howard Jackson.

"At the very beginning of the Rice Code, Miss Narciso went back to the Intensive Care Unit to get a cutdown tray." She had left the Rice Code at approximately 9:36 that evening. At 9:45 the Jackson Code began.

Mrs. Miranda Haber, whose husband was a patient in a room adjoining Jackson's, had testified about the commotion surrounding Jackson's arrest and her recollection that Narciso and Perez had stopped to visit with her at the end of that event. "And she added a wrinkle," Yanko said. "She said that prior to the visit of both nurses, she had observed Miss Narciso alone, walking by [her husband's] room toward Jackson's. They waved to each other." This, Yanko said, had occurred when the hall was quiet, before the commotion began, according to Mrs. Haber.

Those were the basic facts, Yanko said. "Now, why then is Filipina Narciso guilty of murder? "It all begins with the cutdown tray. She had to have a reason for leaving the first Code, however flimsy the reason."

She would not have had to go to the ICU. Others had testified to the availability of a cut-down tray on 4West. That was common knowledge. "So then why did she leave?" She left to go to 5West, Yanko said, first going to the ICU so that someone would remember that she had been there in search of a cut-down tray.

"Why do we say that she went to 5West? We don't. Mrs. Haber does. And what was she doing there, ladies and gentlemen? What was she doing—walking down a dead end corridor where there was no exit when there was an emergency going on down below her at the time she left?" She had not stopped to speak with Mrs. Haber, only waved.

Mr. Murphy had spoken of seeing nurses in and out of Mr. Jackson's room the night he died but could not describe all of them. "There exists the possibility," said Yanko, "that Mr. Murphy saw Filipina Narciso."

Yanko continued, speaking of each arrest and the conflicts and contradictions in the testimony the jury had heard. Although the prosecution had no obligation to present a motive, as Delonis had said, Yanko did speak of the defendants' references to the problems resulting from understaffing. Then he said, "We contend and ask you to find that the evidence does show beyond a reasonable doubt [that the defendants are guilty of the charges against them] and that together they formed a alliance, a conspiracy with the intent to injure."

But there was ambivalence, he said. The women had conspired to injure, on the one hand, but to avoid death on the other. "If you really wanted to kill someone, you wouldn't go out of your way to ensure discovery." To undertake poisonings in the ICU was like trying to drown someone in a pool surrounded by lifeguards, but that was what the women had done. In almost every case they had had reason to believe that the arresting patient would be found in distress. "On each occasion an alarm had been set. On one occasion it didn't go off."

And so Filipina Narciso was guilty of the murder of Howard Jackson. "Although her purpose was not to kill, she knew the consequences of acting with a dangerous drug. —She intended willfully to do the act, and she knew full well the natural and probable consequences of doing that act.

"Ladies and gentlemen, I indicated to you awhile ago that there were forty-three reasons which point to guilt. There is a forty-fourth." The forty-fourth was a combination of all the forty-three, he said. "What are the odds, what is the chance, what is the probability that these defendants have engaged in these activities and that all these factors that are incriminating could exist and the defendants would still nevertheless be innocent?

"Leonora Perez and Filipina Narciso are guilty of the crimes of which they are accused."

CHAPTER 64

"This process you are about to begin is one of the most fascinating in the whole American system of justice because it operates in absolute secret.

We will never know the reason for your decision. —If you come back with a one-word verdict, it is deafening. And if you come back with two words, it is freedom."

It was Tuesday morning. O'Brien stood facing the jury, beginning his closing statement for the defense. There was no mistaking the intensity in his voice. Gone was the relaxed, conversational tone that had characterized his approach to the jurors during much of the trial. His face was solemn now. There was noting relaxed about his posture.

He spoke first about the presumption of innocence, then about the principle of reasonable doubt, saying, "[A]ny doubt, any single, solitary doubt based upon reason is sufficient in and of itself for you to—come back and say 'Not guilty.'"

An individual on trial in a serious matter is at a great disadvantage, he said, especially when faced with the enormous power and resources of the federal government. "The power to accuse in this country is an enormous power. There are many people who are willing to believe that because a person is charged, they are guilty. You weren't selected in this case because you believe that, obviously. —You all said 'No,' I don't think just because [the defendants] are sitting over at that table, that that in any way implicates them in this case. But you can test yourselves on that." They had heard testimony in the case in which other people had been placed in circumstances that were identical to ones they had heard about concerning the two defendants. "[A]nd I wonder if you weighed them in the same way. You have to be careful."

"There is another reason you have to be very careful in this case, and that is because it is a circumstantial case." The chance of a miscarriage of justice increased in a case based on circumstantial evidence. "[T]he chance that you can convict innocent people increases. It has to, because you don't have any direct proof.

"You didn't hear of one criminal act that either one of these women committed, not one." There was no evidence that either defendant had had Pavulon in her possession. Neither had been seen giving an injection to one of the arresting patients. "What if they [the FBI] had found a syringe with a fingerprint of one of these women on it? Would we have a different case? Of course we would."

A case based on circumstantial evidence depended on inference and speculation, he said. In the case of Bart Martin, "the testimony is that Miss Narciso went up to the patient, told him to have a nice dinner and left. Is it possible to infer from that that she gave him an injection?"

The only patient who had a memory of his arrest had to be called by the defense, "and he comes in and he says the last person [in his room] was a man in green. Now what does that tell you about the government's theory? That it doesn't fly."

The prosecution wanted the jurors to infer or guess or speculate, "You can't do that. You don't guess away somebody's freedom.

"What I see going on here, and it troubles me, is selective focus, that when it's two Filipinos, it means one thing and when it's somebody else it means another."

These were women who had never been in trouble, had never even had a traffic ticket. They had been excellent nurses, were trusted even since the indictment. The government could provide no motive for their actions. "So is it likely or probable that they go around killing patients? No, it's not.—So be careful as you look at these circumstances. Just don't rush to judgement."

O'Brien spoke of the women's Filipino background and the fact that English was not their first language. Thus, there had been room for misunderstanding when the two were interrogated. What would it have been like to be in a room with an FBI agent for six hours?, he asked.

Then he turned to the murder charged to Narciso. Why had the prosecution not called Max Murphy to testify even though he was the most compelling factual witness at the trial? "Maybe Mr. Yanko, when he gets back up again in his rebuttal tomorrow, will give you some reasonable explanation as to why Mr. Murphy wasn't called as a witness." Mr. Murphy had telephoned the FBI within weeks of the experience, O'Brien said, because he was troubled by what he had seen.

The prosecution claimed there was a ten-minute period during which Miss Narciso left the Rice Code and went to 5West to murder Mr. Jackson. During that same period Mr. Murphy had seen a man in Mr. Jackson's room stroking his IV line. "Are we to believe that [Miss Narciso] walked past Mrs. Haber and, having seen her and waved, decided she's going to go in and murder the man [in the adjoining room] though she knows there's a witness that's seen her?"

And as to the man seen stroking Mr. Jackson's IV line, "What does she do? Push him away? Hold him off, and at the same time give [Jackson] a fatal injection, then leave the room undetected and unseen?"

This was absurd, O'Brien said. "Doesn't it take more than that to convict somebody of first degree murder?"

No one had seen Miss Narciso in the room. No one saw her give an injection. "I don't know how you can infer—that she, beyond any doubt based upon reason, is guilty of the crime.

"I don't want to spend a lot more time on this cutdown tray because I hope you can see it's a phony issue. —No one ever said there *was* a cut-down tray in the utility room on 4West. They said that's where you *might* find one. No one said there *was* one there." And, as O'Brien reminded the jurors, it was hospital policy that an ICU nurse was responsible for bringing a cut-down tray to an emergency.

He followed by enumerating a number of instances in which other individuals might be suspected based on the same sort of circumstantial evidence. "But they [the prosecutors] tell you as to these other people who were in similar circumstances, who were with patients five minutes before the Code, disregard it.—It was Lippy's depression that caused the man in green to develop. It is a harmless thing when it comes to Earline Fuller [being in Berry's room before he arrested]. We are not to be concerned about that, don't bother about that, put that out of your mind. That should give you no doubt at all.

"Why did the government agents say they didn't want to hear about the man in green [in Lippy's room]?" Bonnie Bates Weston had testified to seeing a man dressed in green leaving the CCU a few minutes before Jordan Olson's Code. "[D]on't be concerned about that, the government says, that shouldn't give you any reasonable doubt."

One by one O'Brien spoke of the charges against Narciso, claiming repeatedly that there was nothing but proximity to involve her in the patients' arrests. "So if you look at each one of those, something is missing and it comes down to this: the sum is not greater than its parts."

Yanko had asked them to run all the charges together. But the fallacy in that, O'Brien repeated, was selective focus. "What about these other people?"

The FBI agents had not been geared up to go into the hospital and say they couldn't solve the problem. That was not an option open to them, O'Brien said. "They go in and solve crimes. —They say if this isn't the answer then you can come up with a better one.

"I say to you today, in this courtroom, isn't it the time for us to do that? Maybe it will happen in a different way."

O'Brien seemed about to conclude, but then he went on. The day before he had seen a young woman holding a small child in the hall outside the courtroom. She had been looking for the room where new citizens were sworn in, he said. Doubtless she had been told what it would be like to be a citizen with all the great protections the country provided.

"Don't you understand?" They were a jury that had agreed to be honest and fair, he said, not to prejudge a case or speculate, guess, or conjecture. This was the protection the country's law provided.

"I hope that when [Miss Narciso] was told that 'You're 29, your life is at an end, you will disgrace your family and friends,' I hope that when Mrs. Perez was told she wouldn't see her children again, that those people weren't right. I hope they were wrong."

The emotion O'Brien brought to these closing words was unmistakable. During the recess that followed the spectators in the courtroom were unusually quiet. After so many weeks and so many words, O'Brien had summoned up the stark reality in a very few, the future facing the nurses should the jury find them guilty.

CHAPTER 65

When the jurors returned to the courtroom, it was Edward Stein's turn to speak for the defense. He approached the podium, patted his sheaf of notes into place, and began to speak, addressing the jury in a mild, almost conversational manner, one as different from his earlier manner as O'Brien's had been.

They were in an artificial situation, he said, a situation in which the communication was all one way. He would speak. They would remain silent, unable to ask questions, and this was a situation that could lead to misunderstandings. "It would be so much better if we could sit down where we felt comfortable, over a cup of coffee, over a beer, and talk about these things. But we can't do that. We have to do it this way."

He paused. "You're about to make a big decision. I don't think any of us has ever made a bigger decision than you will make very soon.

"It's important to Leonie and P.I. because the rest of their lives depend on it. It's important to this country because you can reaffirm—the principle set down 201 years ago. It is important to the world. The world is watching.

"And it's important to you members of the Jury. You're going to have to live with your decision, each of you, for the rest of your lives and that may be the sternest test."

It was the government's obligation to prove beyond a reasonable doubt that each patient listed in the indictment had received an injection of Pavulon, that this was a purposeful criminal act, and that one or both women had performed that act.

In the cases of Lenz, Olson, and Lippy the government had proved beyond a reasonable doubt that these patients had received Pavulon, Stein said. As proof there was Dr. Anne Hill's testing and he FDA's discovery of the drug in the patients' urine. But in the cases of Martin, Mercer, and Berry there was no such proof, no nerve stimulator test, no antidote, no FDA testing of urine. "Maybe they got Pavulon, but maybe they didn't," Stein said. The physicians treating these patients had testified that they did not know the cause of the arrests. The paid experts the prosecution had called to testify had never examined the patients. They gave opinions about the presence of Pavulon, but doctors' opinions are not infallible.

Stein turned now to what he termed a third group—Howard Jackson and Sheldon Rose. Jackson had been a very sick man, Stein said, a man with failing kidneys and an infection in his bloodstream that was out of control, problems that could have been the cause of his death. Had the FBI laboratory in Washington really found Pavulon in his exhumed tissue? "No one else in the world has ever extracted Pavulon from human tissue," Stein said. There had been no validation of FBI testing procedures at an independent laboratory, although such validation was a minimum requirement for acceptance in the scientific community.

(Stein did not mention that Roger Aaron had provided the defense with tissue samples and a detailed description of the procedures he had followed so that the attorneys could obtain such validation from an independent laboratory. Apparently they had, but they did not made the report public in court.)

Sheldon Rose's treating physician had admitted that Rose had possibly suffered a heart attack. "Doesn't that make you wonder about Mr. Rose?," Stein asked. Didn't it provide room for reasonable doubt?

Having provided reasons to question Pavulon as the cause of the arrests in the second and third groups of patients, Stein turned to the counts charged against Leonora Perez. He began with Homer Mercer's arrest. The only evidence in this case, he said, was the uncorroborated testimony of Mercer's son. No one had heard the son cry out that his father wasn't breathing as he said he had. "Maybe he didn't scream it, maybe he just thought it," Stein said. "But, more importantly, was that person in white [beside Mercer's bed] Leonora Perez?" Mr. Mercer's son didn't know her at the time, didn't know her name, and there was no indication that he knew her by sight. He was confused about the identity of the doctor who had told him his father might not pull through. "A face-to-face conversation. You don't forget who you were talking to in 12 to 15 hours unless you are under enormous stress. How much more shaky can the identification be?

"But the government says, 'That's okay, that's proof beyond a reasonable doubt and if it's a little weak, don't worry about it. This is only reason 16 or 23 or 41. Remember reason 44, the combination, the big picture.'" Reminding them that Judge Pratt had instructed them to look at each count separately, Stein continued.

The prosecution said it was not going to put blinders on the jurors, was going to prove every fact. But what had occurred?, he asked. He spoke of witnesses not called by the prosecution, notably Robert Lippy and Max Murphy, both of whom had important memories that would not have aided the prosecutors' case. Referring to Lippy, he said, "I know he was the only victim with any memory at all. I know that from August, 1975 on he told the FBI that the last person in his room was a man in green. —Whatever else is jumbled in his mind, that's been clear." Weren't the jurors entitled to know that?

It was fortunate that the defense lawyers had interviewed Lippy and called him to testify, Stein said, fortunate that they were able to put Max Murphy on the stand.

Stein gestured toward Dr. Lindenauer, who was sitting in the courtroom. What is he doing here?, Stein asked. He's head of a four-hundred-bed hospital containing many sick people. "What the hell is he doing here today? He's here because he's helping to get a conviction." He had been interviewing doctors before they testified, Stein said. He had tried to extract a confession from Filipina Narciso. He had offered a bribe for testimony. Why wasn't he on the witness stand?"

The VA administration, the FBI, and the government attorneys were trying to wrap up a neat package, solve the problem and put it away, Stein said.

"So you're presented with a conspiracy, two people. Yanko had asked the day before, 'how dark could be the soul of one who could do these acts?'" But these women had been respectable, caring, well-liked people all their lives. Suddenly they had dark souls? "Come on," Stein said.

"How did it [the conspiracy] start? Did they go into the Conference room in the ICU for dinner one night and one says to the other, 'I'm not hungry, let's go out and poison people'?" Did that seem probable? "What is the motive?"

The judge would tell them that the prosecution didn't have to prove a motive, but maybe the lawyers had been hinting at one. Yanko had said the women didn't want the patients to die, just wanted to cause them pain and agony. "How come? As a protest against understaffing? Is that what he was hinting at?"

Mrs. Perez was accused of poisoning Arthur Lenz. She had supposedly shooed his wife and sister out of his room and somehow managed to inject Lenz with Pavulon. But Mrs. Perez had denied even being in the room when those women were there. And the accounts given by Mrs. Lenz and Mrs. Mason had contained contradictions and internal inconsistencies, and they did not agree with others' testimony about the event.

"Doesn't that compel you to conclude that Mrs. Lenz and Mrs. Mason are just mixing things up? But the government says, 'Oh no, this is corroborated. This time we've got somebody else [to corroborate what Lenz and Mason said]. Bonnie Bates Weston. Bonnie Bates 'Immunity' Weston."

Weston had been interviewed ten or twelve times by the FBI about the events of August 15, particularly about the Lenz Code, and had never mentioned seeing Perez alone in Lenz's room. She testified before the grand jury that she had seen Perez and another nurse in the room. Now at trial, twenty-one months later, she recalled seeing Perez alone.

Bonnie Bates Weston had been a suspect in the case, having been several times in situations that could raise suspicion. She had reason to be worried, and so she and her lawyer had struck a deal with the prosecution and she received immunity. "Must have seemed like Christmas." Stein smiled. "Bonnie Bates Weston received immunity. What did the Government receive in return?"

Robert Lippy's mother's testimony was confused at best and had been contradicted by Lippy himself. "And what about this man in green?," Stein asked.

His tone grew more challenging as he spoke of the FBI's methods of interrogation, of the government attorneys' efforts to trip Perez up during their examination. But they couldn't trip her up, he said, because she was telling the truth.

Not one member of the hospital staff had ever seen either nurse mistreat a patient or do anything that appeared suspicious. Witness after witness had testified to the women's good characters. "Leonie Perez must not be convicted on the issue of speculation and conjecture that the government has presented to you," Stein said.

"Very soon—your deliberations will start. —Very soon the trial will be over. And you will finally be able to go back to your families, go back to your lives—walk away from this building. And you will walk away from this case. But I promise you, this case will never leave you. You'll remember this case forever, you will remember Leonie and you will remember P.I.

"Their future depends on your decision, and in large measure yours does, too. You want to be comfortable with your verdict.

"And I'm done. My closing talk is done."

Then, leaving the podium, he took a step or two toward the jury box, his voice dropping to a whisper. "I have just two more words to say to you. They are the last words you will hear from me, and I wish and I beg and I pray that they are the first two words I hear from you: Not guilty."

CHAPTER 66

On Wednesday, the twenty-ninth of June, Judge Pratt was expected to give his final instructions to the jurors before they began deliberations. More than one hundred spectators were crowded into the second-floor courtroom, waiting to hear the judge speak, but before that happened Yanko would address the jury once more to rebut the defense attorneys' closing arguments.

When he took the podium, he was quick to attack those arguments. They contained many innuendoes, he said, many veiled accusations. Although he had tried to present the facts in the case, the defense had not really discussed the facts. "What was discussed, ladies and gentlemen, had to do—with putting blinders over your eyes and I'd like to speak to that."

In their presentation of the facts, Yanko said, the defense attorneys had engaged in "a very clever, selective distortion of the truth." In their comments about the presumption of innocence, they had irresponsibly maligned others. He intended to address each of these comments. "And if I should miss one or two—you'll have to chalk it up to the fact that I finished my task at twenty-five to five this morning, which is when I left my office."

Yanko took on the defense's arguments point by point. He rebutted much that the attorneys had said about expert witness testimony and the FBI lab's testing. Then he turned to the attorneys' arguments regarding individual patients. Was it really understandable that Filipina Narciso had forgotten so many details in the cases of Martin and Rose?, he asked. Was the testimony given by Homer Mercer's son really so questionable?

O'Brien had asked whether Narciso would be likely to pass in the corridor and wave to Mrs. Haber if she was on her way to kill Howard Jackson. But people were walking around the hospital all the time, waving to other people, Yanko said. A nurse doing this would not seem suspicious. Why would Narciso worry about being seen?

He spoke of Robert Lippy and the man in green. "I suggested to you the other day that—you would be well-advised to disregard [his] testimony. Not because it doesn't fit the government's theory of the case but because—Mr. Lippy, in testifying before you, discredited himself." Then Yanko went on to slightly modify what he had said. "If you want to believe Robert Lippy, believe him. Consider everything that he has said and if you want to believe [him], believe him."

Concerning the Sheldon Rose event, said Yanko, the question was why Narciso had not asked a nurses' assistant to go from the ICU to the fourth floor for the needed IV solution but instead had gone herself. O'Brien had suggested that Miss Narciso didn't treat people like "gofers." Yanko shrugged. "Well, perhaps that explains it," he said drily.

He spoke of the contradictory testimony Perez had given with regard to Jordan Olson's arrest. He spoke of the defense attorneys' claim that the FBI agents had threatened the nurses during heavy-handed interrogations, which two agents had strongly denied. He spoke of Bonnie Bates Weston and the grant of immunity. "Reference [was made] yesterday to buying her testimony." But, he said, the jurors might consider why the government would buy the testimony of an individual whose basic testimony on two events had been corroborated.

In returning their verdict, the jurors needed to concern themselves with the credibility of other witnesses' testimony as it conflicted with that of the defendants, he said, and proceeded to list nineteen such witnesses.

"Ladies and gentlemen, you have heard the Defense. What is the defense based on facts? When I was in law school I had a prof who had a favorite saying. —It was a catchy little phrase and this prof had a way of repeating it: 'Nemo Dat Qui Non Habet.' The phrase seemed appropriate at that moment, Yanko said, because it referred to the defense (and the absence of facts). 'Nemo Dat Qui Non Habet' was translated "He who hath not cannot give.'"

* * *

At two o'clock that afternoon, following a break for lunch, the court reconvened. The spectators watched expectantly as Judge Pratt entered, impressive as always in his black robes. He began his instructions to the jurors by cautioning them that they must "reach a just verdict regardless of the consequences. The question is not will the government win or lose. The government always wins when justice is done whether the verdict is guilty or not guilty."

He then proceeded to read the entire indictment against the nurses. The jurors' task was to reach a unanimous decision on each separate count, he said.

He spoke of the difference between direct, hard-fact, eyewitness evidence and circumstantial evidence based on inferences drawn from fact. Each separate inference must flow from proven fact, he said, not from another inference. An inference was more than suspicion, conjecture, or speculation. It was a deduction or conclusion that reason would permit to be drawn from certain facts.

"The law does not permit your decision to be swayed by sympathy, bias or public opinion. It is your sworn duty that if these defendants are not guilty beyond a reasonable doubt that you vindicate them."

When he had finished speaking, the jury rose to leave the courtroom. All eyes were on them as they walked single-file toward the door, six men and ten women, such familiar faces now. Daily from nine in the morning until five in the afternoon they would meet in a guarded jury room to deliberate until they had reached a verdict. Nights they would be sequestered in a nearby Detroit hotel under the guard of federal marshals.

Of the sixteen impaneled, four had been selected at random to serve as alternates. They would be sequestered apart from the other twelve, and would have no part in deciding a verdict unless one of the twelve were for some reason unable to continue to serve.

Perez and Narciso left the courtroom shortly after the jury, refusing to talk to reporters. The defense lawyers declined to discuss the case as well, though in response to a reporter's question Stein turned and said, "You want to know what it's like to sweat out a verdict in a case like this? I'll tell you what it's like. It's scary. Just scary as hell."

CHAPTER 67

Judge Pratt had ordered the defendants and all the lawyers in the case to remain within ten minutes of the courtroom while the deliberations were in progress. Accordingly, all settled in nearby hotels and prepared to wait.

Yanko had told reporters that he did not expect the jury's deliberations to be lengthy, but in fact before a verdict was reached the deliberations set a record for a criminal trial at the Detroit federal courthouse.

Reporters camped in the hall outside Judge Pratt's court, turning the space into a sort of makeshift press room. They passed the time reading, rehashing the evidence, or playing game after game of backgammon while they waited for any sign that a verdict was imminent. On the Fourth of July they had waited almost a week.

If a light were turned on in the courtroom, the reporters hurried to see whether the jury had returned. Any federal marshal leaving the vicinity of the jury room was swarmed. As the days went on, the reporters sometimes caught a glimpse of three or four jurors, dressed in shorts or jeans, doing exercises in the courtroom as though it were a gym, evidently needing the exercise.

One day the reporters spied a brown envelope handed through the jury room door into the keeping of a federal marshal and were certain this indicated that a verdict was forthcoming, but no announcement followed. It seems likely that the envelope contained a note from the jury to Judge Pratt, requesting clarification of his instructions. At any rate, Judge Pratt received such a note on the seventh day of deliberations, asking that he clarify his instructions regarding the single murder count. The jurors had apparently been questioning the concept of premeditation.

Quickly Pratt called the court into session. In the presence of the jury, the defendants, and the attorneys for both sides, he reread the murder count, then explained once again the criteria that must be met for a murder conviction. The jurors must find that poison was used and the act was premeditated and committed with malice and forethought before they could return a guilty verdict.

Now, after the jury left the room, Yanko objected. Although in his closing argument he had suggested that the defendants did not intend to kill patients, he now contended that the use of poison to kill indicated premeditation.

Pratt disagreed. Pavulon was not arsenic, he said. It was not a recognized poison but rather a drug used therapeutically in the operating room. "This is not the usual case of poisoning," he said. "It cannot be inferred from a finding of Pavulon as the poison that the act was premeditated" or that murder was intended.

As the jury's deliberations entered a second week without a verdict, Judge Pratt ordered the jurors to begin working longer hours. The original nine-to-five schedule was extended to include deliberations from seven-thirty to nine-thirty in the evening. After their dinners, the jurors were to return to the muggy jury room for another two hours of deliberation.

O'Brien later wrote, "The days passed without a word. The longer the jury stayed out the more we worried. Now it was almost two weeks since the jury had started deliberating."

During these weeks Dr. Lindenauer was besieged with calls from the media wanting information and statements about the ongoing deliberations. He recalled, "One evening our family was sitting at the dinner table when the phone rang. Susie [his ten-year-old daughter] ran to answer. When she came back I asked who'd called. She said, 'He said his name was Walter Cronkite, but I told him you couldn't talk. You were having dinner.'" Startled, the family laughed.

Cronkite had begun opening his *CBS News* broadcasts by saying, "It's Day Four in the Filipino nurses' case—Day Five, Day Six, Day Seven." Newspapers began computing the number of hours the jury had deliberated and what it was costing the government, estimating that lodging, meals, security arrangements, and jury pay amounted to $2,100 a day. But still there was no verdict.

"On the morning of July 13," O'Brien wrote, "I sat with the nurses in their hotel room. A game show was playing on the television. Suddenly, a banner was flashed on the lower portion of the screen announcing that the jury had a verdict in the Veterans' Hospital case. Moments later, we received a call to come to court."

The courthouse was electric with excitement when they arrived. Cameras flashed. Reporters jostled in the halls. Friends and family stood, tense and silent, waiting to enter the courtroom.

O'Brien wrote, "The jury looked somber as they took their seats. The spectator section was jammed, the first row occupied by correspondents from each of the networks, the wire services, and the nation's major daily newspapers. Then the foreman [of the jury] rose, and the clerk called the first count. There was not a sound in the courtroom."

After ninety-four hours of deliberation, after more than fifteen days of waiting, the moment had come. The defendants and their lawyers stood motionless. The foreman squared his shoulders and looked toward Judge Pratt. In the stillness, the word he spoke was like a hammer blow. "Guilty," he said.

"A low but perceptible moan went through the spectator section," O'Brien wrote. "The clerk [read] the remaining charges. By the time he finished, the women had each been convicted of three counts of poisoning. Miss Narciso was acquitted of one count of murder and one poisoning count." Both were found guilty of conspiracy.

"We were stunned and exhausted," he wrote. "We had worked seven days a week, twelve hours a day, for more than a year. —We had tried to do everything right, but somehow it had not worked."

The prosecutors were exhausted, too. The scope of the case they had presented at trial was enormous. They had faced skepticism, protest, and outright hostility, and they, too, had worked long days for many months. Their success had been purchased at a price.

After the verdict was announced, the women were led from the courtroom and ushered into an anteroom nearby. The attorneys for both sides appeared at news conferences, facing crowds of eager reporters.

Speaking for the prosecution, Yanko declared that all along he had felt confident of a conviction. Asked by a reporter whether the convictions meant that Perez and Narciso had been involved in all fifty-eight breathing arrests that had occurred at the VA in 1975, he replied, "All we're concerned with at this time and all the defendants stand guilty of are those events that were tried." But he added, "One could conclude that all those events were perpetrated by the same individual or individuals."

A few minutes later O'Brien told reporters that the defense attorneys were devastated, saying he could not believe that on the thin and scanty evidence presented any jury in its right mind could convict the women. Voice shaking, he called the verdict unjust and the jury unfair. "Rest assured we plan to appeal," he said.

Together with their attorneys and family members, the women left the courthouse. Faces tear streaked and somber, they shoved past the waiting cameramen and reporters. They were to remain free on bond overnight but were to appear in court once again the next morning at which time Judge Pratt would decide whether or not to continue the bond and would set a date for sentencing.

The prosecutors had said they were undecided about whether or not they would seek the maximum sentence. The defense attorneys declared that they intended to file motions for a mistrial and a directed verdict of acquittal.

But all that lay in the future. On this hot summer day, Leonie Perez and P.I. Narciso were on their way home. For the first time in weeks they would sleep in their own beds if, for them, sleep was possible.

PART 3

THE AFTERMATH

CHAPTER 68

A storm of protest was not long in coming. On the afternoon the verdict was announced, members of the Philippine Nurses Association met outside the courthouse to demonstrate against the jury's decision. A spokeswoman for the group declared, "We registered nurses are not going to take this kind of verdict." It would affect international relations around the world, she said.

In the Philippines the news was met with "utter dismay," as reported on the *Voice of the Philippines.* The Philippine embassy in Washington called into question the United States' system of justice, as did Pacifico Marcos, the younger brother of the Philippine president. He was "disappointed," he said, in a system that relied so heavily on circumstantial evidence.

At the VA hospital anger and outrage were intense. "Any nurse who stays here is risking professional suicide," one nurse was quoted as saying. Another declared that she was taking no chances answering Codes if being near an arresting patient could involve her in a murder charge. There was talk of resignations.

In the next few days 8,500 members of the Michigan Nurses Association would call for a congressional investigation into the convictions. Local churches would begin to circulate petitions in support of Perez and Narciso. The *Ann Arbor News* would soon be flooded with letters protesting the verdict.

But on the night the verdict was announced, the two women gathered with friends and family to pray. They spoke by telephone with an interviewer from the *Detroit Free Press,* saying they had little hope of escaping long jail terms despite the appeals their lawyers intended to file. They could hardly believe what had happened, they said. Perez declared she had lost faith in the American system of justice. "All my faith is gone. I know I did not get a fair trial." She thought the jury had not been fair, that she and Narciso had been discriminated against. She called it racial prejudice, a claim that would be voiced repeatedly in the days ahead. She was afraid for her family, she said, should she be sent to jail. "I'm thinking so much of my two boys. —If I do go to jail they will have no future."

The few jurors who consented to speak with the press in the next several days said that, although they were exhausted and drained, they felt they had made the right decision. Not so the alternates, who had had no voice in that decision. Two who were interviewed expressed dismay. They had felt that the jurors were leaning toward acquittal when deliberations began, they said, but, because they were not included in the deliberations, they did not know what had changed in the jury room.

How the jury had reached a guilty verdict was, some months later, the subject of an article in the *Ann Arbor Observer*, a monthly paper distributed locally. A reporter for the paper had managed to find three jurors who, having taken part in the deliberations, were willing to discuss them.

The jurors had come from diverse backgrounds, they said, but they got along well. In the beginning they had disagreed about the question of guilt or innocence, with some feeling that Narciso and Perez were innocent victims of FBI harassment. Others felt that they were probably guilty but questioned whether the proof against them was substantial enough. Still others were undecided.

The deliberations began with an effort to decide whether Pavulon had in fact caused the patients' arrests. This was not a difficult decision. More difficult was deciding whether the prosecution's contention that the drug would have had to be injected two or three minutes before a patient's arrest by someone nearby was plausible. And much depended on its plausibility. The jury spent two days going over medical testimony on that issue, finally rejecting the defense arguments for the possibility of a delayed effect.

Then, methodically, one by one, using charts and a blackboard, they began to go through the testimony related to each arrest. The three jurors interviewed insisted that they had not taken any witness at his or her word but had studied each witness's testimony very carefully. Gradually they began to see that these various testimonies fit together tightly but were repeatedly contradicted by what the defendants had said.

Under their lawyers' gentle questioning, the women had made a favorable impression on the jurors, but when cross-examination began, that changed. There were so many conflicts, so many inconsistencies and contradictions. "When Ms. Perez denied she was even in Homer Mercer's room at the time his son saw her there, I almost fell off my chair," said one of the jurors being interviewed.

In time the jurors became convinced that the defendants were lying, and lying repeatedly, in an attempt to mislead the jury.

In the case of Bart Martin's arrest, the jurors did not believe Narciso's version of events. Medical records indicated that Martin had an IV line in place at the time of his arrest, though Narciso claimed the line had been discontinued. And it was difficult to believe that someone other than Narciso had time to slip into the CCU and inject Martin in the two and a half minutes that elapsed after she left the unit, someone unnoticed by the nurses' assistant in the room at the time.

The jurors never seriously considered this nurses' assistant as a suspect. They felt there was no other evidence to place her under suspicion. But her presence in the room did seem to fit the prosecution's argument that the defendants had aimed for patients in distress to be discovered in time to call a Code.

At this point the jurors began to realize that no one but Narciso could have poisoned Martin, and they became emotional. They didn't want to find her guilty.

They continued, carefully going over each of the remaining counts until one day a juror suddenly said that something had been bothering her throughout the trial. She had to speak of it.

The deliberations halted while the woman explained that before she was selected as a juror she had seen a newspaper article reporting that a woman named Betty Jakim had claimed responsibility for the poisonings, At once the jurors began a search of the trial record for mention of Jakim, but they found insufficient information to make her a serious suspect.

Similarly, in spite of the defense argument that there were a number of other possible suspects, none seemed sufficiently plausible. One or both of the defendants *had* been at the victims' bedsides within two and a half minutes of the poisonings. But perhaps what weighed most heavily was the jurors' belief that Narciso and Perez had been lying in their testimony. This, taken together with the other evidence, led to a conclusion of guilt beyond a reasonable doubt.

CHAPTER 69

Early on July 14, Perez, Narciso, and their attorneys set out once again to drive to Detroit for an appearance before Judge Pratt. The road stretched out in the morning sunlight. The women sat silent, not knowing whether the judge would allow them to remain free on bond or would order them jailed that day.

Again they were greeted by a throng of well-wishers milling outside the courthouse. Many more were crowded into the courtroom, some wearing blue ribbons pinned to their chests as tokens of support.

The hearing began promptly. The prosecution was quick to ask that the women be jailed at once. They had been convicted of crimes "too horrible to be contemplated," attorney Delonis declared. If left free on bond, they could flee to their homeland, out of reach of US law.

Judge Pratt rejected the request, saying that the women would remain free on bond while their conviction was being appealed. He saw no indication that they would flee. They could have done so months earlier and had not. As to sentencing, he said that he would impose a sentence after he received a report from the women's probation officers, a report that could take a month to six weeks to prepare.

The defense attorneys would appeal the conviction as soon as the women were sentenced, O'Brien told reporters. They would take the appeal as far as it had to go. "If that means all the way to the Supreme Court, we'll do it," he said. In the meantime, the defense would file a motion for retrial based on the government attorneys' abuse of the grand jury system and would file a motion for directed acquittal.

The women had won a small victory that day. When they left the courthouse, they wore no handcuffs or other restraints.

★ ★ ★

The day before, directly after the verdict was announced, Dr. Lindenauer had closed the hospital to the press, ordering that no employee or staff member was to be interviewed within the building. This appeared prudent given the disruptions in hospital routine resulting from the relentless presence of reporters in the early days of the investigation. But now access to the hospital seemed less important. There was news to be gleaned without entering the building.

The *Detroit News* reported that a source interviewed at the courthouse claimed that the jurors were hurt by O'Brien's criticism of their verdict, the women jurors in particular. According to the source, "He was their darling."

Robert Lippy, who had never thought the nurses were guilty, maintained this belief. He would help them any way he could, he told an interviewer. If he had to go door to door asking for donations to pay for their defense, he would do it.

Reporters learned that a rally was planned on the grounds outside the

VA. There would be speakers, including the convicted nurses. If permission to hold the rally on hospital grounds were denied, the rally would be held someplace nearby, an organizer declared, but on a Sunday in September some eight hundred people were massed on the hospital lawn, more overflowing onto land across the road.

It was a field day for reporters. The crowd chanted and sang. Little Christopher Perez marched through the throng carrying a sign almost as big as he was, which read, "Mommy and Auntie P.I. are innocent."

A number of nurses in uniform marched as well and with them a scattering of patients in pajamas and robes. A petition to Judge Pratt, asking for a new trial, was passed hand to hand for signatures. The rally's organizers urged the crowd to send letters protesting the verdict to President Carter and Michigan congressmen. Already nurses from the University of Michigan Health System had telegraphed the president expressing shock and concern.

One of the alternate jurors spoke to the crowd, calling the verdict a miscarriage of justice. A former patient who had been cared for by Narciso spoke of how she had comforted him when he couldn't sleep. "Now she's being slapped on the butt," he said.

When, at length, Perez and Narciso stood up to speak, the crowd roared. "On the thirteenth day of July justice died," Narciso told them. "I don't know how many more innocent people will be convicted. I hate to think that some day one of you will be in our shoes."

Perez repeated that she had lost faith in the US judicial system. "But I have high hopes that justice will come out and truth will prevail in this country."

Both women were eloquent, surprisingly so. The difficulty they had had expressing themselves when questioned on the witness stand was no longer apparent. But here they were not defending themselves. Here they were surrounded by some eight hundred people who firmly believed in their innocence.

Yet belief in the women's innocence left a large question unanswered. If Perez and Narciso were not guilty of the poisonings, who was? It seems likely that this question was on the minds of many of those working in the hospital that summer. Doctors were watchful, alert to any event that might be considered suspicious.

On July 7, while the jury was still engaged in deliberations, a patient on the hospital's fifth floor had begun to have difficulty breathing. On orders from Dr. Lindenauer, the doctor in charge of the resuscitation had specimens collected and taken to a laboratory for testing in case the results should be needed for evidence in court. Although the testing turned up no evidence of a drug not ordered for the patient, the very fact that specimens were collected is an indication of the level of unease in the hospital. "I grabbed specimens and asked questions later," the doctor said.

Among the nurses, apprehension was widespread for another reason. They feared that their mere presence at a Code could involve them in an accusation of murder. That possibility no longer seemed far-fetched. It had happened to P.I. and Leonie.

As the summer wore on, demonstrations in support of the women took place in neighboring communities. Fund-raising events proliferated. Letters poured into the *Ann Arbor News* claiming that the women had been framed, that they were scapegoats because of their ethnic background, while a scattering complained about the cost to the taxpayers of the lengthy investigation and trials. One of these suggested deporting both women to the Philippines to save taxpayers the cost of their incarceration.

CHAPTER 70

Late in August Judge Pratt set a date for sentencing. The women were to appear before him at 2:00 p.m. on the fifteenth of September.

September 15 was a dreary day. Before noon a crowd had gathered outside the courthouse, huddling in the rain, holding rain-streaked placards protesting the nurses' conviction. Inside the building security was stringent. Judge Pratt had ordered the upper floors sealed until shortly before the hearing began, and then only those holding passes would be admitted above the first floor. Clearly the judge anticipated an unwieldy crowd.

Perez and Narciso entered the building in the early afternoon. Their lawyers went directly to Judge Pratt's chambers to hear his decision before it was announced in court. "We don't know what to expect," O'Brien told reporters. "All we can do is hope for the best." But, he added, that because he believed in the women's innocence, he thought any sentence would be unfair.

Shortly after two o'clock the women and their lawyers entered the hushed courtroom. They stood motionless before the judge while he announced what they had already learned: the sentencing would be delayed. Before he passed a final sentence, Pratt was ordering Narciso and Perez to report to the Federal Reformatory for Women at Alderson, West Virginia, where, for as many as ninety days, they would undergo psychological evaluations. After prison officials gave him a report on these evaluations, the women would return to Detroit for sentencing. He was ordering the evaluation, he said, "because of the nature of the case and its complexities." He did not elaborate, and in less than fifteen minutes the hearing ended.

Although Judge Pratt had received a long and detailed report from the women's probation officers, he evidently wanted more information. Speaking later to reporters, Delonis claimed that the judge's decision was not uncommon. A presentencing report could not go into the kind of depth that a psychological evaluation could. Stein agreed that the decision was not unusual. "It's common when you have a case like this where nothing fits," he said, adding once again that the women had unblemished records and the crimes for which they were convicted were very much at odds with their natures.

The following Thursday Perez and Narciso set out for West Virginia accompanied by an assortment of family members and friends and, in addition, the Philippine consul general from Chicago, who was present, he said, to provide "moral support." There were no federal marshals in the entourage. Judge Pratt had ruled that the women could travel on their own but would travel at their own expense.

They were met by the warden of the reformatory. He reported that the women seemed tired from the journey and rather apprehensive. "But," he said, "I think they were somewhat relieved—when they saw the place here was more like a college campus, and not surrounded by high fences or guard towers."

Alderson was a minimum-security prison with a single maximum-security unit reserved for inmates who were considered dangerous. On the day Narciso and Perez arrived, there were only four inmates in this unit, all women accused of threatening assassinations of US presidents. The other inmates lived in low brick cottages and had private rooms to which they were given keys. There were no bars on the windows. There were no prison uniforms. And yet, despite the absence of barred windows and guard towers, Alderson was a prison, and for as many as ninety days, Perez and Narciso would be prisoners there.

While the women were accustoming themselves to their new circumstances, their lawyers were filing motions. One motion asked Judge Pratt to set aside the jury's verdict and declare the women not guilty. The defense attorneys argued that the evidence the prosecution had presented was insufficient to permit any reasonable juror to find them guilty. A second motion requested a new trial. The third requested the determination of a mistrial. Both of these motions claimed that improper conduct by the prosecutors had hurt the women's right to a *fair* trial. The mistrial motion claimed, further, that the jurors had acted improperly in discussing newspaper reports regarding Betty Jakim, as the *Ann Arbor Observer* article had mentioned them doing. The jurors had been ordered by Judge Pratt to consider only the evidence presented at trial, and they had disregarded that order. This was grounds for a mistrial ruling, the defense motion argued, as was attorney Yanko's earlier statement to the press claiming that he would know the defendants were guilty regardless of the jury's verdict.

If either of the latter two motions were granted, the government could decide to prosecute again, whereas a grant of acquittal would leave the women free and no longer subject to prosecution on the same charges. Clearly a grant of acquittal was what the defense hoped for.

Delonis responded to the defense attorneys' efforts in a written legal argument tinged with anger. The defense was blaming the nurses' conviction on "their oft-played allegation of prosecutorial misconduct," he wrote, "and on a newer theme of juror misconduct during deliberation." It was not grounds for a mistrial, Delonis argued, that the jury should allude to the articles about Betty Jakim when the defense, during trial, had itself made reference to her.

Hearings on the motions were scheduled for October.

By the time these hearings were under way, the evaluations at Alderson were coming to a close. The nurses had spent only five weeks in the facility when Judge Pratt received a report on the doctors' findings. "We're expecting to hear something [about the women's release] from the warden tomorrow," O'Brien told reporters in early November. "The girls should be home shortly."

On the fifth of November Perez and Narciso were released. Now, again, they would wait to learn Judge Pratt's decision.

CHAPTER 71

The decision was more than a month in coming. But on the morning of December 19, in a ruling that stunned the prosecutors and left the defense attorneys jubilant, Judge Pratt ordered a new trial for Narciso and Perez, saying that a new trial was merited because "the interests of justice and judicial conscience demand it."

In granting the new trial, Pratt laid responsibility for his order entirely at the feet of the two government attorneys who had tried the case, citing Delonis and Yanko as guilty of "numerous improprieties." The attorneys had kept the defense "off-balance" by withholding evidence and redacting important paragraphs from FBI reports that would be favorable to the defense. This was a tactic, Pratt said, "that subverts the trial from a search for truth to a game of five-card stud poker." The list of prosecution witnesses had been changed after the trial began, making it difficult for the defense to focus on a single strategy. The material had been released in a piecemeal fashion right up to the final weeks before the trial and into the trial itself. This made a "mockery" of the government's earlier promise to follow an "open-file" policy in the case, Pratt said. "The right to a fair trial necessarily includes within it adequate notice and opportunity to prepare." The prosecution had repeatedly failed to comply with the court's orders to release pretrial information to the defense.

Prosecution attorneys had made improper statements to the press. They had been improper in their questioning before the jury and had persisted in this line of questioning even when it was ruled improper. The overwhelming prejudice to the defendants arising from the government's misconduct prevented the jurors from receiving the case free of taint, Pratt said.

In addition, he said, the prosecution's case was entirely circumstantial. The government had submitted no direct proof of guilt on any count. "Plainly enough the case against the defendants was not overwhelming," he said, concluding that "the insidious accretion of Prosecutorial misconduct in this case polluted the waters of justice as surely as if the prosecutors had argued that the jurors should ignore the dictates of the Constitution."

The granting of a new trial was not an acquittal. Judge Pratt's ruling had not declared the women innocent, but the news of a new trial was greeted jubilation. "It's a terrific Christmas present," O'Brien told reporters, and Narciso agreed. In a voice shaking with emotion, she said, "This will be the first good Christmas for us in three years."

There was a champagne party that night, held at one of Ann Arbor's venerable taverns. The women celebrated with their families and friends, Perez cradling her smallest son in her arms all evening. But the possibility of another trial still lay ahead. O'Brien said, "My only regret is that these women may have to go through all this again."

Many believed that the government would be reluctant to try the case again. Judge Pratt's ruling had discredited its case to such a degree that it was questionable whether a new trial based on the same evidence would have any chance of succeeding. But this was only speculation. What the government would decide remained to be seen.

* * *

During the last days of the trial, a new US attorney had been sworn in. James K. Robinson took office after the jury had announced its verdict, after posttrial motions had been filed, and only a short time before Judge Pratt granted a new trial.

Robinson was a man in his early thirties. Although he had done criminal defense work, he had no experience as a federal prosecutor. Now, suddenly, he was confronted with an enormous responsibility. As a US attorney he was obliged to decide whether the government would reprosecute or dismiss the case against the nurses. He said later, in discussing the decision, that the case was the first "really hot potato" delivered to him in his legal career. "I had to decide what to do, and I had to do it in the climate of very public attention."

In a memorandum written after he had reached his decision, Robinson explained his reasons for making the determination. He began, he said, by carefully assessing what success the government could expect to have in retrying the case. The likelihood of convictions had been decreased, he believed, by the reduced number of charges that would be presented at a new trial. Originally there had been eleven alleged victims, now that number had been reduced to six. The jury had acquitted on some counts. Judge Pratt had ruled out others. Robinson felt that a jury might conclude that the nurses' presence at these few arrests was only coincidence.

In addition, the prosecution's evidence was, and would continue to be, entirely circumstantial. There were no witnesses to say they had seen the women giving injections. And, while the government was not obliged to prove motive, the fact that there was none was "a huge, huge problem," Robinson wrote. Besides, there was the need to overcome great skepticism concerning the women's guilt that had been displayed by both the public and the press since the indictments in 1976. That two women with no prior criminal or antisocial background could have conspired to carry out such a bizarre plan seemed hardly credible.

Of paramount importance was the question of whether proceeding with a new trial would "promote the ends of justice, instill respect for the law and advance the course of ordered liberty," Robinson wrote. Given the reduced likelihood of procuring convictions in a new trial, acquittals would confirm for many the belief that the first verdict had been obtained solely through prosecutorial misconduct and would undermine faith in the criminal justice system in America. "Clearly, this had an impact on the decision to dismiss," Robinson said. "And that was my decision, made with the help of others."

The trial prosecutors vigorously disagreed with the decision, feeling strongly that the government should retry the case. The FBI concurred. In fact, as Robinson recalls, the FBI "took me 'upstairs' to Washington to the Criminal Division [of the Department of Justice]" to argue against his decision to dismiss the case, but there the deputy assistant attorney general sustained the decision.

On the first of February, Narciso and Perez stood with their lawyers in the federal courthouse, hearing Judge Pratt grant the prosecution's motion to dismiss all charges against them. And so the long ordeal ended. They could not be tried again on the same charges. They were free.

Shouts of joy rang through the hospital when the news reached Ann Arbor. "I almost keeled over when I heard my friends wouldn't have to go through it again," said one VA nurse. But not everyone was convinced that the dismissal was the right decision. Another nurse commenting on the women's future, said that the fact that they hadn't been found innocent in a court of law was a problem. To start doing something with their lives would be "rough," he said. They would have a hard time finding a job because every "run of the mill" person on the street would think they got off on a technicality.

As the reactions to the government's decision continued, celebration was mixed with puzzlement. If the nurses were innocent, who was guilty? Should the government have pursued the investigation, looking for an answer to that question? Official reaction was muted. The hospital administration refused to comment.

In the Philippines news of the dismissed charges was welcomed, but a newspaper there raised questions, asking who would compensate the nurses for the indignities they had suffered. "Can these two nurses ever again obtain decent employment in any American hospital after the damage done by publicity to their persons? Will American patients trust them with their lives again?"

It was a question Narciso and Perez were asking themselves. Both had expressed a desire to return to nursing in the United States, but whether this would be possible was in question. Whether there were hospitals that would hire them was uncertain. Whether their applications for US citizenship would be denied was uncertain as well.

Following the judgment for dismissal, the women were able to travel again outside the limited confines of Michigan. That summer they returned to the Philippines for a brief stay. They received a hero's welcome there. Dinners were held in their honor. Leonie Perez's hometown organized a parade. The two spoke at universities, hospitals, and churches, thanking those who had helped raise $85,000 for their defense. But many Filipinos were disappointed to learn that the women had decided to proceed with their applications for American citizenship and wondered why they would want to return to a country where they had been treated so badly. Narciso answered, saying that what had happened to them did not involve all the American people, that many had supported them.

And so later that summer they returned to Michigan to look for jobs. According to O'Brien, several hospitals and private clinics in the area had expressed interest in hiring them, some operated by Filipino Americans, some not.

* * *

In Ann Arbor the VA hospital was confronting lawsuits. Seven civil damage suits had been brought by victims' families, of which four had been settled. Others were pending.

There was a general feeling of exhaustion in the building. The fever of excitement surrounding the trial and its aftermath had faded, leaving only weariness in its wake. Routines continued as they always had. Breakfast trays rattled into patients' rooms. Doctors filed, white coated, through the halls. Blood pressures were taken, temperatures recorded. Visitors arrived bearing potted plants and magazines and candy.

Most of the nurses who had spoken of resigning had not done so. Even some who had been particularly hostile to the hospital administration remained on the job. Patients crowded the outpatient clinics. Residents complained of lack of sleep. The hospital was returning to normal.

CHAPTER 72

Early in 1980 Leonora Perez and Filipina Narciso became citizens of the United States. By then both had been working for some time in hospitals in the Detroit area.

As O'Brien had earlier predicted, neither seems to have encountered difficulties in obtaining nursing positions. In an interview with the *Detroit Free Press*, Perez is quoted as saying, "The assistant director [at the hospital where she found work], he ask me, 'We want you to come to work, when you want to start?' So I have no problems." Apparently Narciso had a similar experience at another hospital near Detroit and claimed to be happy in her new position.

The women are in their sixties now. Narciso continues to live and work near Detroit. In 2008 she received an award from the Daisy Foundation, an organization that honors excellence in nursing in hospitals nationwide. Leonora Perez is an RN at the Camp Pendleton Naval Hospital in Southern California and is the mother of three grown sons.

That both women have pursued successful careers in the years since the trial must be a source of great satisfaction, but inevitably that ordeal will have marked their lives. To spend months confronting the specter of life imprisonment and to face the horror of the jury's verdict cannot have failed to leave scars. Whether the pain of these memories has diminished in the intervening years is a question for Leonora Perez's youngest son to answer.

Jason Magabo Perez, a graduate with a master of fine arts degree from University of California, San Diego, has undertaken to write a novel about the court case involving his mother, a case he believes was filled with false accusations and manipulated evidence. He calls doing this a challenging experience. Speaking with his mother about her fears and anxieties was not something the family had done to any extent. The novel has given Jason an excuse to do this.

In the summer of 2009 he gave a public reading of a few chapters from the novel, a reading attended by his mother and a brother. "They loved that their story, fictional sometimes, mattered and people cared," he says.

In fact, many people care. Those who supported the nurses in the 1970s care deeply, believing that the women were insufficiently vindicated by the outcome of the trial. Judge Pratt's decision to call for a new trial was not, after all, an acquittal. The government's failure to retry the case was not a declaration of innocence and, though the women were given their freedom, that freedom came chiefly as a result of prosecutorial improprieties. It was not an exoneration. The jury's verdict was not overturned.

Others, believing strongly in the women's guilt, fault the government for failing to retry the case. That two women convicted of poisoning a number of patients should be set free, suffering no consequences, is a continuing problem for those convinced of their guilt.

These opposing views persist to this day. Judge Pratt's decision is repeatedly questioned. Yet it is difficult to see how he could have decided differently. The United States promises defendants the right to a fair trail when they are accused of wrongdoing. If the fairness of the trial comes into question, the judge must protect the defendant's rights. In *United States of America v. Filipina Narciso and Leonora Perez,* Judge Pratt acted as he was bound to do when he deemed the women's rights had been compromised. He was obliged to see that justice was served as prescribed by the US judicial system, however unsatisfactory this was to his critics.

* * *

Today the old Ann Arbor VA stands in the shadow of a glamorous new neighbor, an immense glass and steel structure built to accommodate the laboratories, outpatient clinics, and other facilities long crowded into the old building. Only inpatients occupy the old hospital now, pushing their walkers through the halls and viewing Tigers games on the television screens above their beds, just as patients were doing thirty-five years ago.

Now, as then, on the first of July a fresh group of young doctors arrives to undertake the patients' care. Sooner or later they will hear about the poisonings, about the killer or killers who once roamed the corridors they hurry through each day. They will hear of the trial of the Filipino nurses and the fear that once haunted the hospital, but for them this will be fading lore, old history soon half forgotten in the rush of their days.

But few who were involved in the long hospital drama claim to have been untouched by the experience. Memories are vivid, emotions still intense. "I don't think anyone who went through it will ever forget what it was like," a doctor told me. "You walk into the hospital one morning and find that someone has tried to murder your patient. That's not something you're likely to forget."

Passing the old hospital one autumn twilight, I remember his words. Lights are shining from patients' windows. Leaves flutter toward the wide front lawn. There is nothing in the tranquil scene to prompt thoughts of the horror once harbored within the building's walls. Yet, for some, there is no forgetting. They will long remember the summer of 1975 when a killer carried death from floor to floor contained in a small syringe.

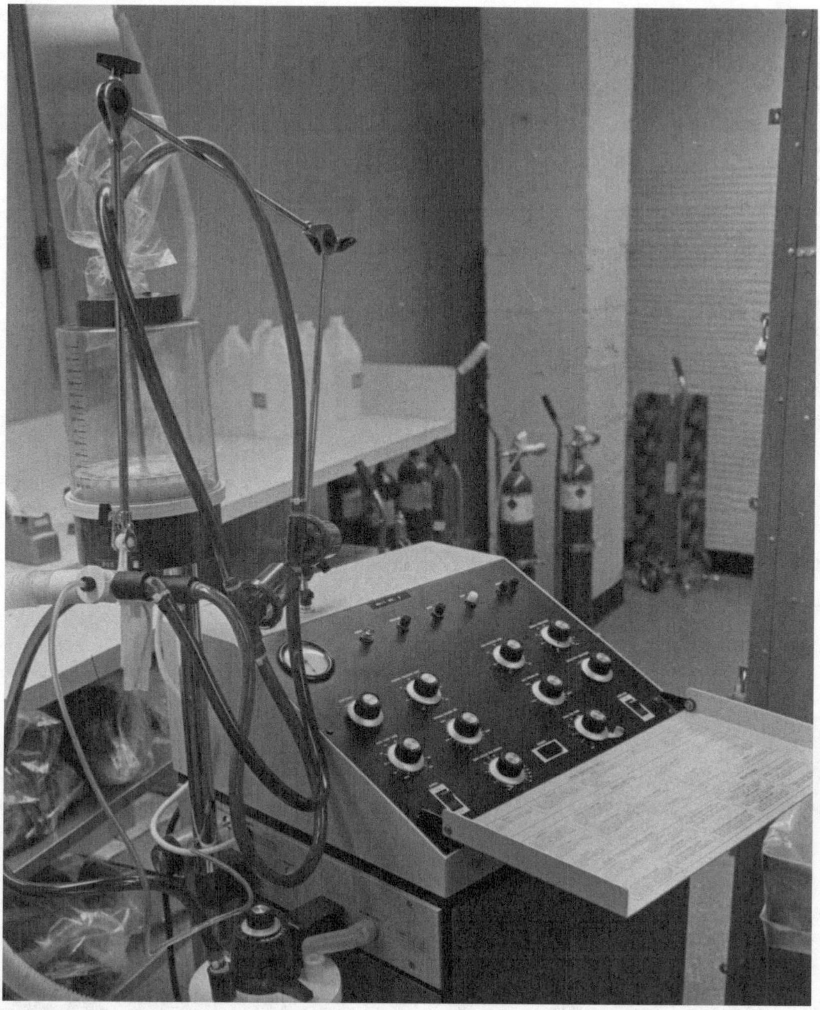

Fig. 1. Respirator machine at the Veterans Administration Hospital, Ann Arbor, September 1975. (© *Ann Arbor News*, September 30, 1975.)

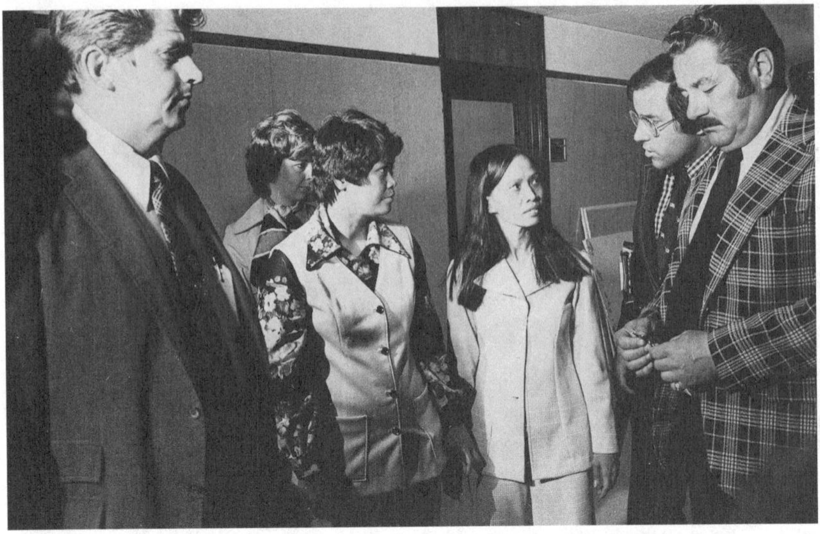

Fig. 2. Felipina B. Narciso and Leonora Perez inside Federal Building after preliminary court hearing, Detroit, July 1976. (© Ann Arbor News, July 1976. Photo by Jack Stubbs.)

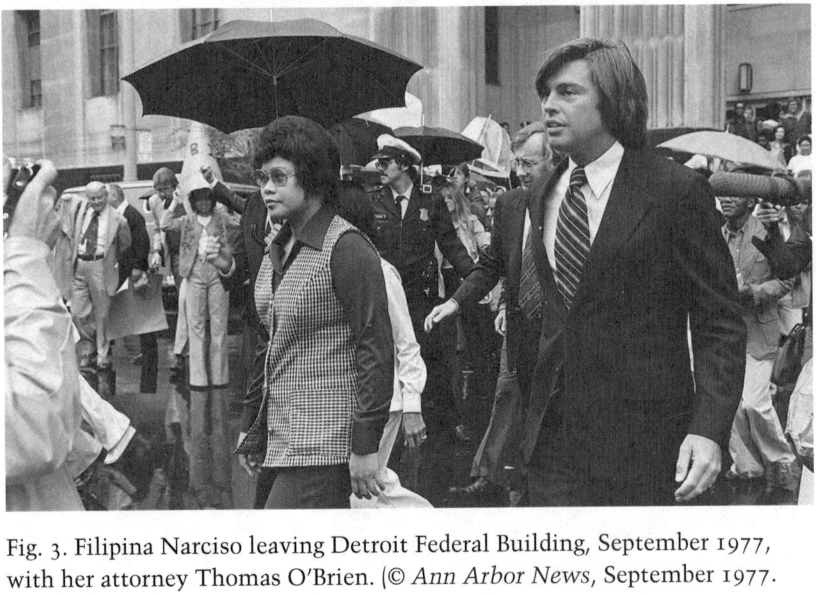

Fig. 3. Filipina Narciso leaving Detroit Federal Building, September 1977, with her attorney Thomas O'Brien. (© *Ann Arbor News*, September 1977. Photo by Jack Stubbs.)

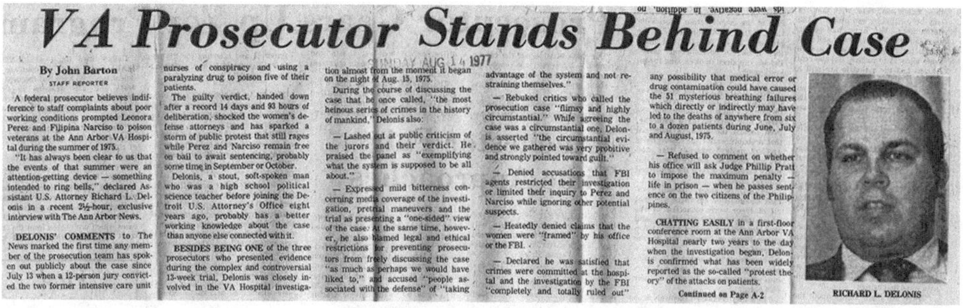

VA Prosecutor Stands Behind Case

SUNDAY AUG 14 1977

By John Barton
STAFF REPORTER

A federal prosecutor believes indifference to staff complaints about poor working conditions prompted Leonora Perez and Filipina Narciso to poison veterans at the Ann Arbor VA Hospital during the summer of 1975.

"It has always been clear to us that the events of that summer were an attention-getting device — something intended to ring bells," declared Assistant U.S. Attorney Richard L. Delonis in a recent 2½-hour, exclusive interview with The Ann Arbor News.

DELONIS' COMMENTS to The News marked the first time any member of the prosecution team has spoken out publicly about the case since July 13 when a 12-person jury convicted the two former intensive care unit nurses of conspiracy and using a paralyzing drug to poison five of their patients.

The guilty verdict, handed down after a record 14 days and 93 hours of deliberation, shocked the women's defense attorneys and has sparked a storm of public protest that still rages while Perez and Narciso remain free on bail to await sentencing, probably some time in September or October.

Delonis, a stout, soft-spoken man who was a high school political science teacher before joining the Detroit U.S. Attorney's Office eight years ago, probably has a better working knowledge about the case than anyone else connected with it.

BESIDES BEING ONE of the three prosecutors who presented evidence during the complex and controversial 13-week trial, Delonis was closely involved in the VA Hospital investigation almost from the moment it began on the night of Aug. 15, 1975.

During the course of discussing the case that he once called, "the most heinous series of crimes in the history of mankind," Delonis also:

— Lashed out at public criticism of the jurors and their verdict. He praised the panel as "exemplifying what the system is supposed to be all about."

— Expressed mild bitterness concerning media coverage of the investigation, pretrial maneuvers and the trial as presenting a "one-sided" view of the case. At the same time, however, he also blamed legal and ethical restrictions for preventing prosecutors from freely discussing the case "as much as perhaps we would have liked to," and accused "people associated with the defense" of "taking advantage of the system and not restraining themselves."

— Rebuked critics who called the prosecution case "flimsy and highly circumstantial." While agreeing the case was a circumstantial one, Delonis asserted "the circumstantial evidence we gathered was very probitive and strongly pointed toward guilt."

— Denied accusations that FBI agents restricted their investigation or limited their inquiry to Perez and Narciso while ignoring other potential suspects.

— Heatedly denied claims that the women were "framed" by his office or the FBI.

— Declared he was satisfied that crimes were committed at the hospital and the investigation by the FBI "completely and totally ruled out" any possibility that medical error or drug contamination could have caused the 51 mysterious breathing failures which directly or indirectly may have led to the deaths of anywhere from six to a dozen patients during June, July and August, 1975.

— Refused to comment on whether his office will ask Judge Phillip Pratt to impose the maximum penalty — life in prison — when he passes sentence on the two citizens of the Philippines.

CHATTING EASILY in a first-floor conference room at the Ann Arbor VA Hospital nearly two years to the day when the investigation began, Delonis confirmed what has been widely reported as the so-called "protest theory" of the attacks on patients.

Continued on Page A-2

RICHARD L. DELONIS

Fig. 4. Lead prosecutor Richard Delonis. (© *Ann Arbor News*, August 14, 1977.)

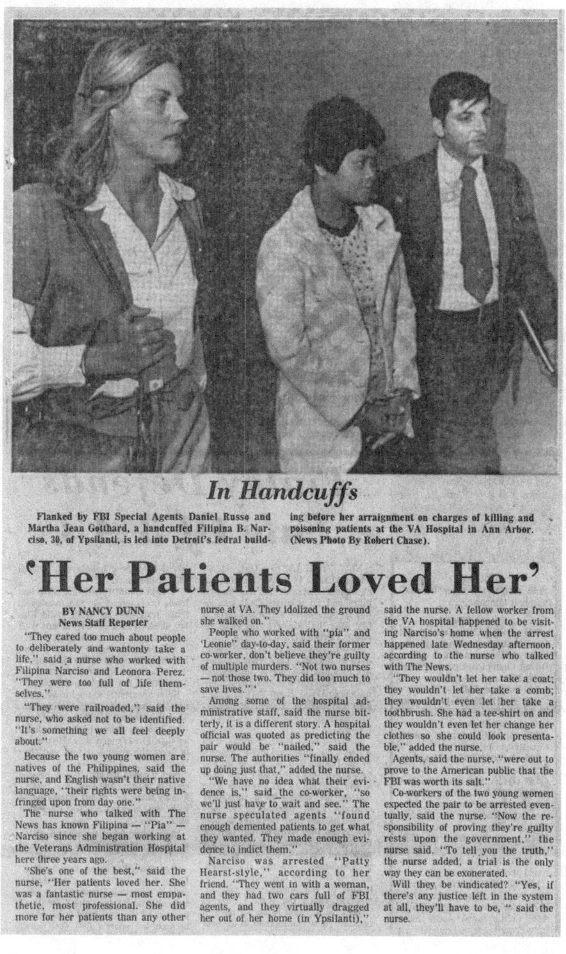

In Handcuffs

Flanked by FBI Special Agents Daniel Russo and Martha Jean Gotthard, a handcuffed Filipina B. Narciso, 30, of Ypsilanti, is led into Detroit's fedral building before her arraignment on charges of killing and poisoning patients at the VA Hospital in Ann Arbor. (News Photo By Robert Chase).

'Her Patients Loved Her'

BY NANCY DUNN
News Staff Reporter

"They cared too much about people to deliberately and wantonly take a life," said a nurse who worked with Filipina Narciso and Leonora Perez. "They were too full of life themselves."

"They were railroaded," said the nurse, who asked not to be identified. "It's something we all feel deeply about."

Because the two young women are natives of the Philippines, said the nurse, and English wasn't their native language, "their rights were being infringed upon from day one."

The nurse who talked with The News has known Filipina — "Pia" — Narciso since she began working at the Veterans Administration Hospital here three years ago.

"She's one of the best," said the nurse, "Her patients loved her. She was a fantastic nurse — most empathetic, most professional. She did more for her patients than any other nurse at VA. They idolized the ground she walked on."

People who worked with "pia" and 'Leonie" day-to-day, said their former co-worker, don't believe they're guilty of multiple murders. "Not two nurses — not those two. They did too much to save lives."

Among some of the hospital administrative staff, said the nurse bitterly, it is a different story. A hospital official was quoted as predicting the pair would be "nailed," said the nurse. The authorities "finally ended up doing just that," added the nurse.

"We have no idea what their evidence is," said the co-worker, "so we'll just have to wait and see." The nurse speculated agents "found enough demented patients to get what they wanted. They made enough evidence to indict them."

Narciso was arrested "Patty Hearst-style," according to her friend. "They went in with a woman, and they had two cars full of FBI agents, and they virtually dragged her out of her home (in Ypsilanti)," said the nurse. A fellow worker from the VA hospital happened to be visiting Narciso's home when the arrest happened late Wednesday afternoon, according to the nurse who talked with The News.

"They wouldn't let her take a coat; they wouldn't let her take a comb; they wouldn't even let her take a toothbrush. She had a tee-shirt on and they wouldn't even let her change her clothes so she could look presentable," added the nurse.

Agents, said the nurse, "were out to prove to the American public that the FBI was worth its salt."

Co-workers of the two young women expected the pair to be arrested eventually, said the nurse. "Now the responsibility of proving they're guilty rests upon the government," the nurse said. "To tell you the truth," the nurse added, a trial is the only way they can be exonerated.

Will they be vindicated? "Yes, if there's any justice left in the system at all, they'll have to be, " said the nurse.

Fig. 5. Felipina Narciso enters the Detroit Federal Building for arraignment with FBI agents Daniel Russo and Martha Jean Gotthard. (© *Ann Arbor News*, July 18, 1976. Photo by Robert Chase.)

VA Jury Request Spurs Conference

WEDNESDAY JUL 6 1977

By John Barton
STAFF REPORTER

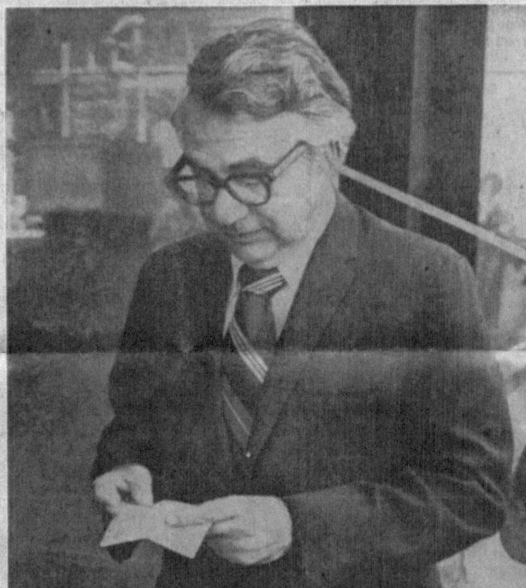

VA Case Judge Philip Pratt Reads Newsclip

DETROIT — Leonora Perez and Filipina Narciso made a surprise appearance in federal court here today as the jury weighing the case against them neared the end of its first week of deliberations.

The two former Ann Arbor VA Hospital nurses were called to Federal Judge Philip Pratt's chambers along with their attorneys for a conference after the jurors requested clarification of an instruction Pratt gave the jury when the three-month-old trial ended.

In a note to the judge late Tuesday, the jurors asked for clarification of Pratt's instruction of the single murder count. Pratt apparently called both sides in to go over the instruction before presenting that clarification to the jury in open court.

The jurors apparently had asked the judge to repeat his instruction for finding a defendant guilty of murder.

PRATT, OVER the objections of prosecution attorneys, said the poisoning in question was not by itself indication of premeditation.

"This is not the usual case of poisoning," Pratt said. "I think it required the government to prove premeditation. It cannot be inferred by the use of the poison in question."

The conference with the defendants, their attorneys and federal prosecutors began shortly before 9 a.m. After the clarification, the jurors filed into the jury room to begin their seventh day of deliberation in the case.

The panel met late into the hot, muggy evening Tuesday, after Pratt ordered an extra two-hour session. Before Tuesday, the panel had met on a 9 a.m. to 5 p.m. schedule.

BY THE END of Tuesday night's session, the jurors had completed 41 hours of discussion without reaching a verdict.

Narciso, appearing calm, was smiling as she entered Pratt's chambers with her lawyers for the closed-door discussion. But she politely refused to talk to reporters.

Perez also refused to speak with newsmen but her husband, Epifanio, said, "We're fine, everything's OK, and we are just waiting like everyone else."

He then asked how long the jury had been out. When informed it was 41 hours he rubbed his hands together nervously and said, "Wow, that is a long time. Were they even out that long for Patty Hearst?"

THE DEFENDANTS, along with close friends and relatives, have spent the past week waiting for a verdict at a downtown hotel.

"She isn't nervous," one of Narciso's friends said, "but I'm a wreck. We didn't think they would be out so long."

Both defense and prosecution lawyers have refused to comment on possible implications of the jury's lengthy deliberations. Perez, 33, of Ann Arbor, is accused of using a paralyzing drug to poison three patients. Narciso, 31, of Ypsilanti, is accused of using the same drug to kill one patient and poison four others.

Fig. 6. Judge Philip Pratt. (© *Ann Arbor News*, July 6, 1977.)

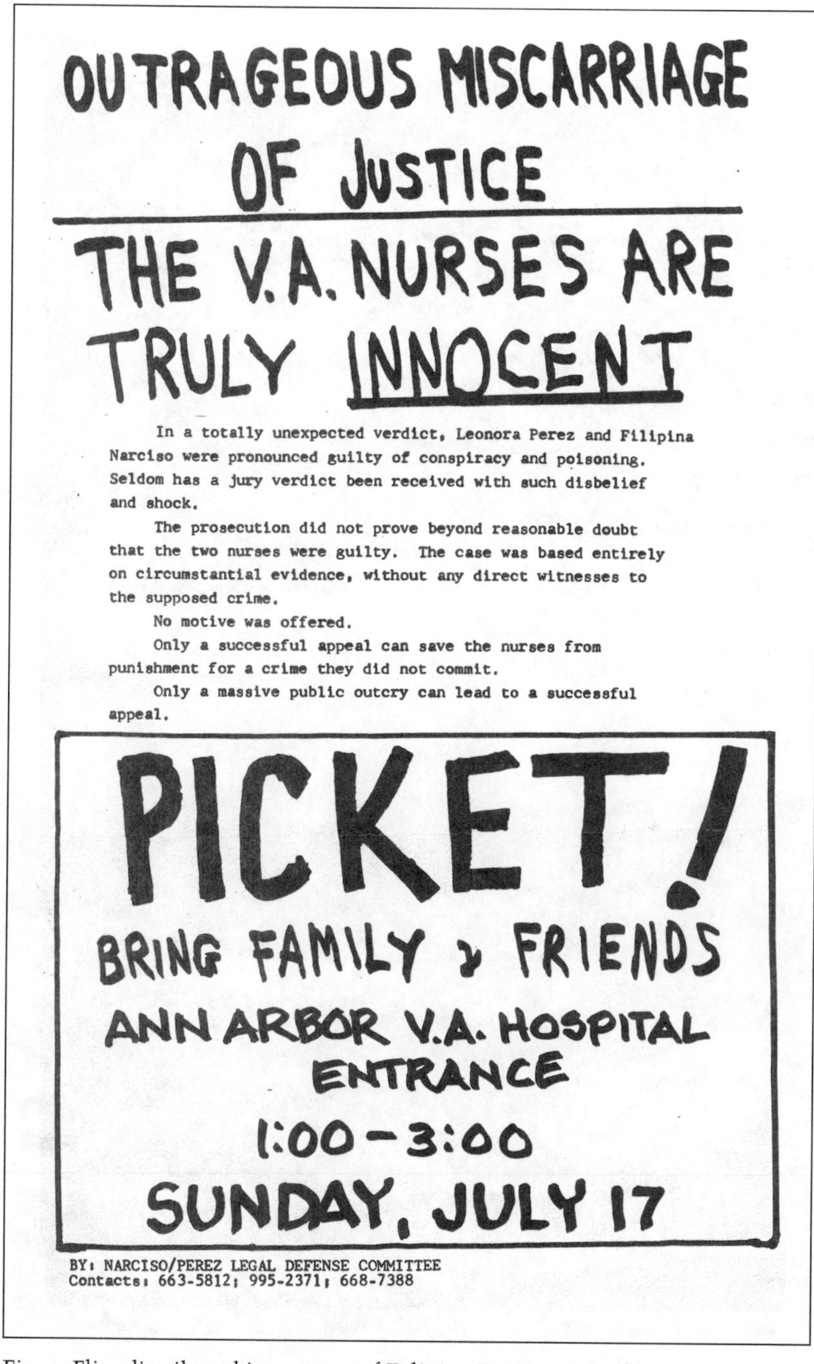

OUTRAGEOUS MISCARRIAGE OF JUSTICE

THE V.A. NURSES ARE TRULY INNOCENT

In a totally unexpected verdict, Leonora Perez and Filipina Narciso were pronounced guilty of conspiracy and poisoning. Seldom has a jury verdict been received with such disbelief and shock.

The prosecution did not prove beyond reasonable doubt that the two nurses were guilty. The case was based entirely on circumstantial evidence, without any direct witnesses to the supposed crime.

No motive was offered.

Only a successful appeal can save the nurses from punishment for a crime they did not commit.

Only a massive public outcry can lead to a successful appeal.

PICKET!

BRING FAMILY & FRIENDS

ANN ARBOR V.A. HOSPITAL ENTRANCE

1:00 – 3:00

SUNDAY, JULY 17

BY: NARCISO/PEREZ LEGAL DEFENSE COMMITTEE
Contacts: 663-5812; 995-2371; 668-7388

Fig. 7. Flier distributed in support of Felipina B. Narciso and Leonora Perez after the nurses were found guilty of conspiracy and poisoning.

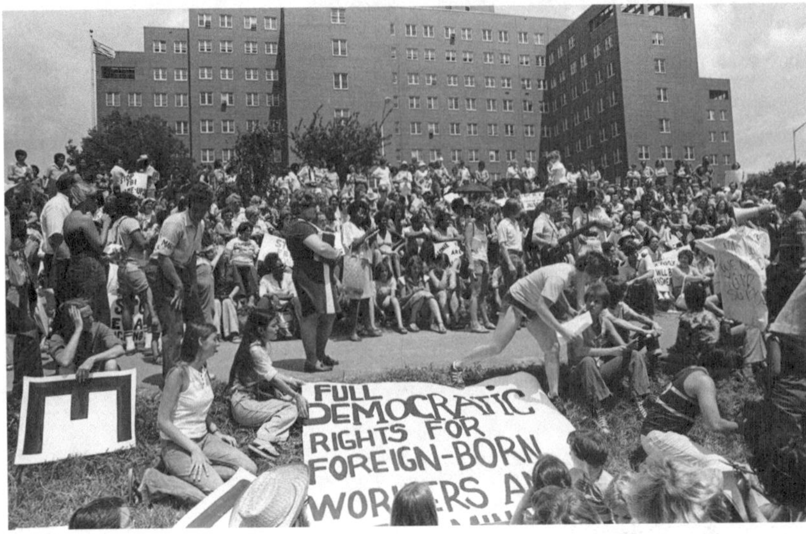

Fig. 8. Crowd estimated at seven hundred persons jam VA Hospital area for protest rally. (© *Ann Arbor News*, July 18, 1977.)

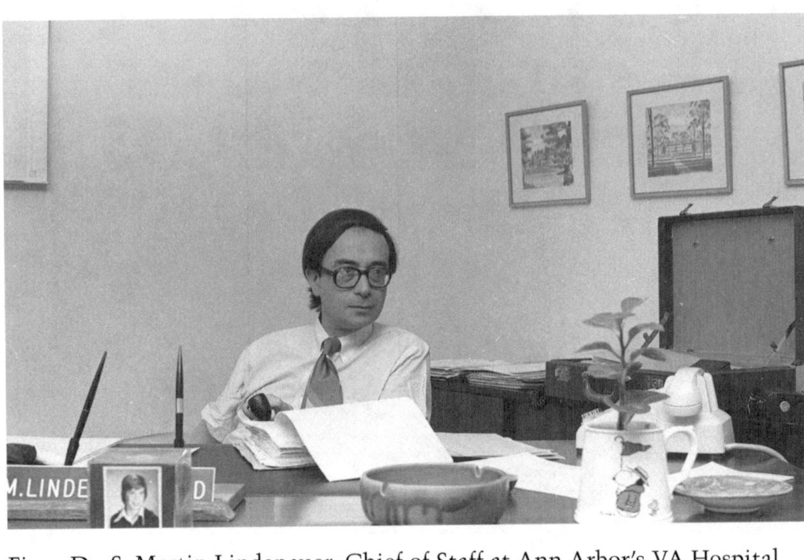

Fig.9. Dr. S. Martin Lindenauer, Chief of Staff at Ann Arbor's VA Hospital. (© *Ann Arbor News*, June 17, 1976. Photo by Cecil Lockard.)

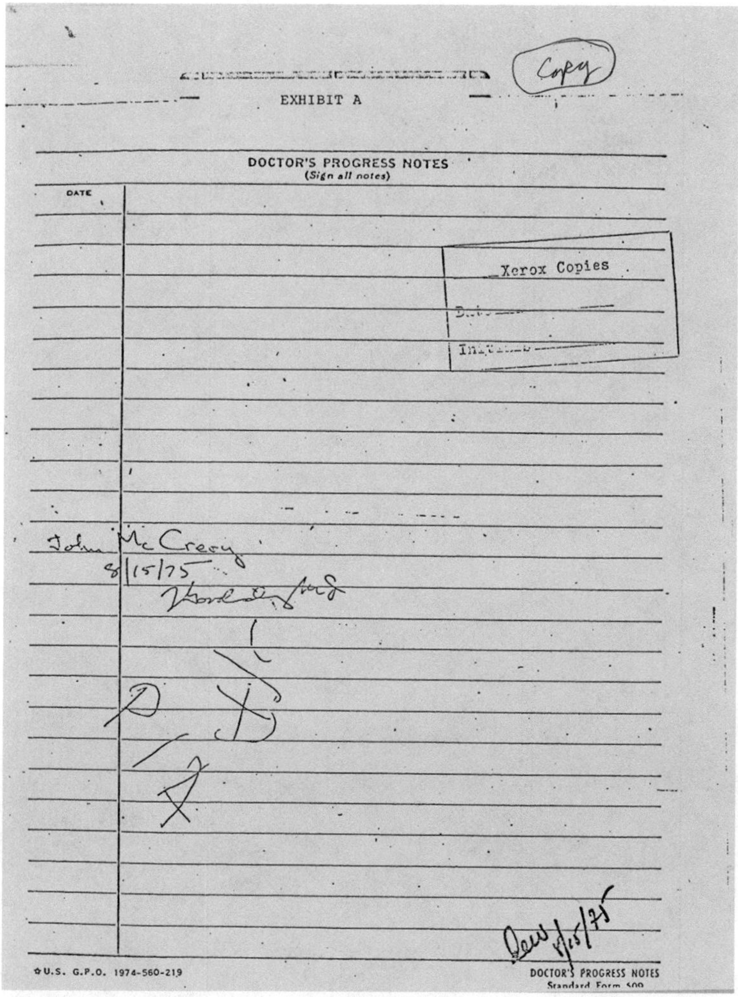

Copy

EXHIBIT A

DOCTOR'S PROGRESS NOTES
(Sign all notes)

DATE

Xerox Copies

John McCrery
8/15/75

☆U.S. G.P.O. 1974-560-219

DOCTOR'S PROGRESS NOTES
Standard Form 509

Fig. 10. John McCrery's written identification of "PIA" as the nurse who had administered medication just before he suffered a breathing arrest, countersigned by Dr. Lucy Goodenday, head of the Cardiology Section.

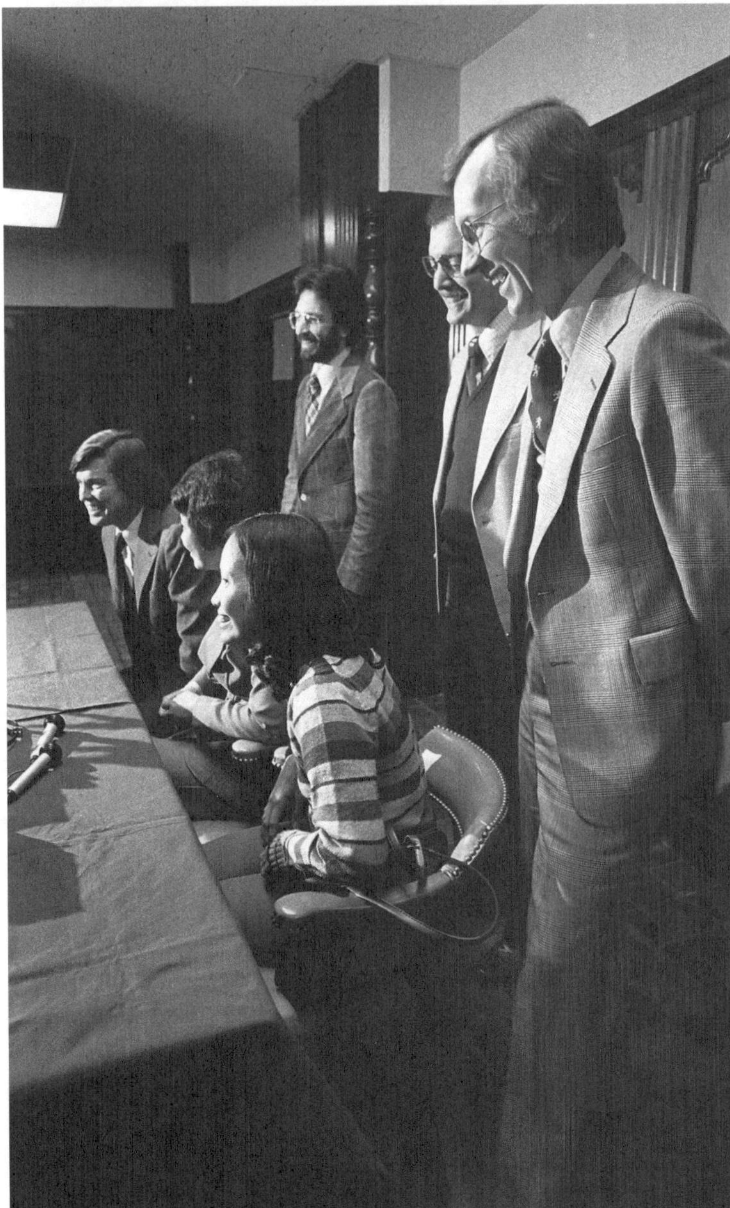

Fig. 11. Filipina Narciso and Leonora Perez with attorney Thomas O'Brien and other lawyers at press conference after charges are dismissed. (© *Ann Arbor News*, February 1977.)

SOURCES AND RESOURCES

Where there are quotes in the text that are not cited below, they derive from personal interviews or transcripts of court testimony.

CHAPTER 1

Free Press, April 15, 1977.
Litigation 11 (1984–85).
Free Press, November 18, 1975.
Ann Arbor News, November 18, 1975.

CHAPTER 3

Nursing supervisor's log, August 1975.
Catherine Cenzina Choy. *Empire of Care*. Durham, NC: Duke University Press 2003, 1.

CHAPTER 5

Nursing supervisor's log, August 1975.
Detroit Free Press, September 4, 1975.
Detroit Free Press, October 19, 1975.

CHAPTER 6

Ann Arbor News, August 12, 1975.
Detroit News, September 5, 1975.

CHAPTER 13

Ypsilanti Press, August 18, 1975.
Detroit Free Press, August 19, 1975.
Detroit Free Press, August 20, 1975.

CHAPTER 14

Ann Arbor News, August 20, 1975.
Ann Arbor News, August 22, 1975.
Ann Arbor News, August 24, 1975.

CHAPTER 15

Ann Arbor News, August 30, 1975.

CHAPTER 17

Ann Arbor News, August 29, 1975.

CHAPTER 19

Ann Arbor News, October 3, 1975.
Litigation 11 (1984–85).

CHAPTER 22

Ann Arbor News, January 13, 1976.
Detroit News, January 14, 1976.
Ann Arbor News, January 14, 1976.
Litigation 11 (1984–85).

CHAPTER 23

Ann Arbor News, May 21, 1976.
Detroit Free Press, May 25, 1976.
Ann Arbor News, June 8, 1976.

CHAPTER 24

Litigation 11 (1984–85).
Ann Arbor News, June 18, 1976.
Ypsilanti Press, August 29, 1976.

CHAPTER 25

Ypsilanti Press, June 17, 1976.
Ypsilanti Press, June 23, 1976.

CHAPTER 26

Detroit Free Press, June 23, 1976.
Ann Arbor News, June 25, 1976.

CHAPTER 27

Ypsilanti Press, June 30, 1976.
Detroit Free Press, August 22, 1976.
Ann Arbor News, August 29, 1976.

CHAPTER 28
Ann Arbor News, September 25, 1976.
Detroit Free Press, October 1, 1976.
Ann Arbor News, October 8, 1976.
Ypsilanti Press, December 29, 1976.

CHAPTER 29
Litigation 11 (1984–85).

CHAPTER 30
Free Press, March 14, 1977
Litigation 11 (1984–85).

CHAPTER 31
Detroit Free Press, March 13, 1977.

CHAPTER 32
Detroit Free Press, March 22, 1977.

CHAPTER 35
Detroit Free Press, March 30, 1977.

CHAPTER 36
Ann Arbor News, March 31, 1977.

CHAPTER 37
Detroit News, April 2, 1977.
Personal journal of Dr. Martin Lindenauer.

CHAPTER 38
Detroit News, April 6, 1977.
Personal journal of Dr. Martin Lindenauer.

CHAPTER 42
Personal journal of Dr. Martin Lindenauer.

CHAPTER 51
Personal journal of Dr. Martin Lindenauer.
Detroit Free Press, May 30, 1977.

CHAPTER 56
Personal journal of Dr. Martin Lindenauer.

CHAPTER 61
Litigation 11 (1984–85).

CHAPTER 62
Personal journal of Dr. Martin Lindenauer.

CHAPTER 68
Litigation 11 (1984–85).
Michigan Daily, July 14, 1977.
Detroit Free Press, July 14, 1977.
Ann Arbor News, July 13, 1977.
Detroit Free Press, July 14, 1977.

CHAPTER 69
Ann Arbor Observer, September 1977.

CHAPTER 70
Detroit Free Press, July 10, 1977.
Detroit Free Press, July 24, 1977.
Michigan Daily, September 15, 1977.

CHAPTER 71
Detroit News, September 16, 1977.
Ann Arbor News, September 23, 1977.
Ann Arbor News, December 20, 1977.
Wayne Law Review 48 (2002–3).
"The V.A. Nurses Case: The Effects of Press Coverage and Public Perception on a High-Profile Trial," 64–65.
Detroit Free Press, February 2, 1978.
James K. Robinson Memorandum, July 22, 1977.
Manila Times Journal, July 1977.

CHAPTER 72
Ann Arbor News, February 3, 1978.

CAST OF CHARACTERS

Aaron, Roger: FBI forensic scientist
Baden, Michael: deputy chief medical examiner in New York City
Bailey, Jay: agent at the FBI's Detroit office
Balls, Lula: nurses' assistant at the Ann Arbor VA hospital (hereafter AAVA)
Barton, John: reporter at the *Ann Arbor News*
Belisario, Mario: chargé d'affaires at the Philippine embassy in Washington, DC
Benner, Jon: resident in the surgery service at the AAVA
Berry, Douglas: patient who suffered a fatal respiratory attack at the AAVA
Bishop, Dr. Ronald: head of the internal medicine service at the AAVA
Brock, Alex: patient who suffered a fatal respiratory attack at the AAVA
Burgess, Laurence: Detroit-based attorney who represented Leonora Perez
Calhoun, Gary: assistant to the chief of the medical service at the AAVA
Chase, Dr. John: chief medical director at the VA Central Office
Cheyfitz, Kirk: reporter at the *Detroit Free Press*
Clark, Daniel: patient who suffered a respiratory attack at the AAVA
Collins, Ian: patient at the AAVA
Custer, Roy: patient who suffered a respiratory attack at the AAVA
Dawson, Robert: assistant director of the AAVA
Delonis, Richard: head of criminal prosecutions in the US Attorney's Office in Detroit
Dyllan, Joseph: patient who suffered a fatal respiratory attack at the AAVA
Feenstra, Phyllis: RN at the AAVA
Foldes, Francis: expert in pharmacology and muscle-relaxing drugs
Foye, Laurence: envoy from VA central office
Freier, Dr. Duane: head of the surgical service and acting chief of staff at the AAVA
Fuller, Earline: nurses' assistant at the AAVA
Gibson, Marilyn: sister of Hannah Wiley, witness to the respiratory attack of

Leonard Meadows
Goodenday, Dr. Lucy: head of the Cardiology Section at the AAVA
Gullickson, Mark: assistant to the director of the AAVA
Gutler, Richard: FBI agent
Haber, Miranda: wife of patient occupying room adjoining Jackson's
Hackett, Barbara: US magistrate who presided over the arraignment of Filipina Narciso and Leonora Perez
Harris, Jonah: patient who suffered a fatal respiratory attack at the AAVA
Hill, Dr. Anne: head of anesthesiology at the AAVA
Hoffman, Marvin: patient at the AAVA
Jackson, Howard: patient who suffered a respiratory arrest AAVA
Jakim, Betty: night nursing supervisor at the AAVA
Kurtz, Dr. Roberta: intern at the AAVA
Lenz, Arthur: patient who suffered a respiratory attack at the AAVA
Lenz, Holly: wife of Arthur Lenz
Lindenauer, Dr. S. Martin: chief of staff at the AAVA
Lippy, Robert: patient who suffered a respiratory attack at the AAVA
Lippy, Verna: wife of Robert Lippy
Marcos, Ferdinand: president of the Philippines
Martin, Bart: patient who suffered respiratory arrest at the AAVA
Mason, Angie: sister of Arthur Lenz
McDougal, Jerrold: patient who suffered a respiratory attack at the AAVA
McLeod, Dr. Michael: surgery intern at the AAVA
Meadows, Leonard: patient who suffered a respiratory attack at the AAVA
Mercer, Homer: patient who suffered a respiratory attack at the AAVA
Moran, Michael: attorney who represented Filipina Narciso
Mourish, Arnold: director of the AAVA
Murphy, Max: patient who occupied room near Jackson's
Narciso, Filipina: RN at the AAVA
Neff, Stuart: patient who suffered a respiratory attack at the AAVA
Nunley, Gloria: chief of nursing at the AAVA
O'Brien, Thomas: Ann Arbor-based attorney who represented Filipina Narciso and Leonora Perez
Olson, Jordan: patient who suffered a respiratory arrest at the AAVA
Orne, Dr. Martin: psychiatrist who testified for the defense
Opstad, Byron: chief pharmacist at the AAVA
Palmer, Rex: patient who suffered a fatal respiratory attack at the AAVA
Penner, Dennis: medical resident at the AAVA
Perez, Jason Magabo: son of Leonora Perez
Perez, Leonora: RN at the AAVA
Pratt, Judge Philip: judge at the Detroit Federal District Court
Rice, Chester: patient at the AAVA

Roberts, Leonard: patient who suffered a respiratory attack at the AAVA
Robinson, James K.: US attorney
Rose, Sheldon: patient who suffered a respiratory attack at the AAVA
Russo, Daniel: FBI agent
Sadasivan, Dr. Kalia: surgical resident at the AAVA
Schaeffer, Raymond: visual information specialist with the FBI
Spiegel, Dr. Herbert: associate clinical professor of psychiatry, College of Physicians and Surgeons, Columbia University
Stein, Edward: Ann Arbor-based attorney who represented Leonora Perez
Stitt, Gordon: patient who suffered a respiratory arrest at the AAVA
Stitt, Hillary: wife of Gordon Stitt
Stross, Dr. Jeoffrey: doctor in the Department of Postgraduate Medicine, University of Michigan Medical School
Sweet, Dr. Robert: chairman of the Department of Anesthesia at the University of Michigan Hospital
Van Dam, Philip: US attorney who replaced Richard Delonis
Wallace, Jeffrey: patient who suffered a respiratory attack at the AAVA
Walters, Milda: analytic chemist at the FDA laboratory in Detroit
Ward, Eugene: first FBI agent to be called to the AAVA
Weatherbee, Lee: chief of pathology at AAVA
Weber, Thomas: resident in surgery at the AAVA
Weg, John: chief of pulmonary medicine, University of Michigan Medical Center
Westbrook, Laurence: assistant US prosecuting attorney–Department of Justice
Weston, Bonnie: nursing assistant ICU
Wiley, Gregory: patient who suffered a respiratory attack at the AAVA
Wiley, Hannah: wife of Gregory Wiley
Wiley, John: chief sample custodian at the FDA
Wiley, Timothy: assistant chief pharmacist at the AAVA
Willock, Dr. Marcelle: anesthesiologist at Roosevelt Hospital in Manhattan and a consultant to the chief medical examiner of New York City
Wilson, Pamela: RN ICU
Wright, Dr. Booker: orthopedic resident at the AAVA
Yanko, Richard: assistant US attorney
Yost, Jerry: patient who suffered a fatal respiratory attack at the AAVA
Zibrak, Joseph: medical intern at the AAVA

ACKNOWLEDGMENTS

Many people helped immeasurably during the preparation of this book. We particularly wish to thank our spouses, Bob Oneal and Marilyn Lindenauer, and our wonderful children for their invaluable support, endless patience, wise counsel, and enthusiastic encouragement. Special appreciation also goes to Cindy Cook, our transcriber extraordinaire, and to Scott Ham, our acquiring editor at the University of Michigan Press, for recognizing the merit of the story and helping us bring it to light with the support of the terrific staff at the University of Michigan.

We also wish to acknowledge the many individuals who impacted and were impacted by the events described in this book. Critical roles were played by Ann Hill, who solved the mystery of the unexplained breathing failures and proved their etiology, as well as by lead FBI agent Dan Russo and his many colleagues and collaborators who persevered in seeking the truth. Less visible but equally important were all of the residents and unnamed members of the medical, nursing, and respiratory therapy staff at the Veterans Administration Hospital at the time, who stayed on the job and continued providing dedicated patient care under extraordinary circumstances. Finally, great appreciation is due to all of the patients and their families, who maintained faith in the care being provided to them and their loved ones during this very trying time.